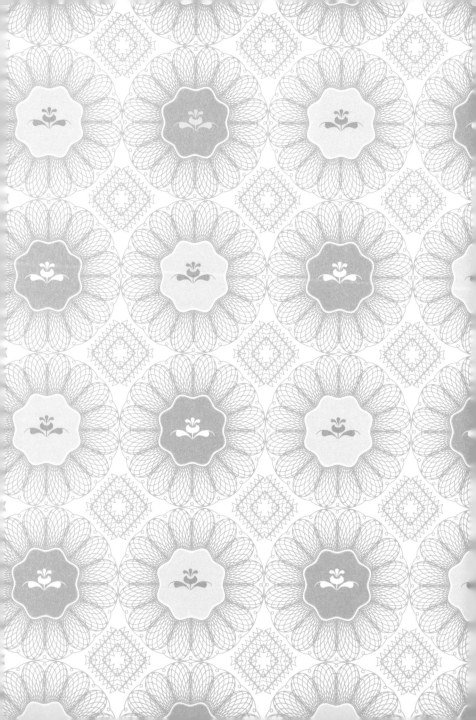

THE BABY VOID

THE BABY VOID

My Quest for Motherhood

JUDITH UYTERLINDE

GUILFORD, CONNECTICUT
AN IMPRINT OF THE GLOBE PEQUOT PRESS

To buy books in quantity for corporate use
or incentives, call **(800) 962–0973**
or e-mail **premiums@GlobePequot.com.**

English translation by Marion Boers
Cover and text design by Georgiana Goodwin

Library of Congress Cataloging-in-Publication Data is available.

ISBN 978-1-59921-296-8

Printed in the United States of America

10 9 8 7 6 5 4 3 2 1

To my brave and strong mother

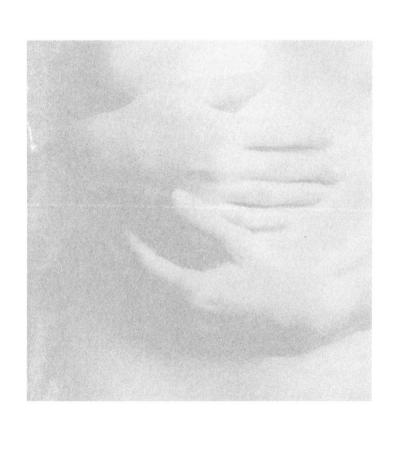

CONTENTS

CHAPTER ONE

THE BEGINNING,

or

How I Lost Twins and My Trust in Psychiatrists

Our handlebars were entwined, although we hadn't even kissed yet. They'd had to push us gently out of the bar after closing time. Now we were outside, untangling our bikes rather clumsily. "May I make an indecent proposal?" he asked. "Would you like to come to my place for another beer?"

I had just met Paul and found him funny and attractive and authentic. All fixed ideas were foreign to him; his thoughts ran wild. He danced in exactly the same uncontrolled manner, with swinging and jerking movements that had something childlike about them. When I saw him dancing, I fell in love.

He lived in a former warehouse, in one enormous room. It was like a refrigerator inside. I would have liked to jump straight into his big bed with him, but I wasn't that bold. I only took my shoes off, as a gesture.

Paul lit the wood stove in the middle of the room. I'd never lit a wood stove before and felt completely out of my league. Perhaps I shouldn't have come. We'd left behind the natural intimacy we shared earlier in the warm bar. Here, he made not a single advance toward the promise of indecency. He did give

2

me a beer; the last he had in the house, he said. I thought I detected a shadow of regret in his voice, but it could just as well have been a hint that I should be moving along. When my glass was empty, I began putting on my shoes and said, rather brusquely, "I'd better go."

The next moment we were standing there, kissing. The rest of the weekend was spent in that big bed, rising only to get something to eat and drink and to put more wood on the fire. The curtains stayed closed, the telephone unplugged. From the scent of our lovemaking, I knew we belonged to one another: We smelled wonderful together. Not that I believed in true love. But from that moment on, I felt every night I spent without him was a night lost.

We walk arm in arm through New Orleans, stopping to listen to every street musician.

"May I make an indecent proposal?" I ask. "Shall we make a baby?"

I want to hear how the question sounds on my tongue. Not crazy, I think. Perhaps it really is a good idea. I figure that having children is part of living. You often hear people say that they love children, or animals. This all-embracing kind of love is unfamiliar to me. I loved my ex's dog, which we took for walks in the forest and on the beach. I love my brother's children, who enjoy coming to stay with us. And I have no doubt that I would also love our child. If I were to have anyone's child, it would have to be Paul's. Idyllic scenes pass before my mind's eye, blended with erotic fantasies: I have our baby on my breast as Paul gently makes love to me.

This sultry, hip-swinging city seems to put me in a romantic flush of insanity. Because, why would someone like me desire children? I want to go on long trips, meet people, party all night, dance and flirt, and learn to play the violin well, and the saxophone, too, if possible. Read all the books in the world, become a publisher, or a writer, or a journalist, or a singer in a rock band. I've never had a pet, and houseplants seldom survive my lack of attention. The role of aunt definitely suits me better than mother. The favorite aunt who brings you exotic gifts from far-off lands. Who tempts you to go with her to the bar before you're actually old enough.

In fact, I had a favorite aunt like that. She smoked and drank lots of wine and chose to remain single and childless. She told me about her complicated relationships with married men. Even though they were always problematic, I found them immensely more interesting and exciting than my parents' married life. I wanted to be like that, too.

If you have children, you automatically become a mother and a spouse. Until now this frightening picture has held me back from the proposal that I am now trying out aloud. I have in the meantime been with Paul for five years. We even share

4

a house, but dull routine hasn't set in yet. A former school friend of mine had parents who—after twenty years of marriage—still acted as if they were in love. They made a game of continually coming up with new pet names for one another. Meanwhile, my parents and most of the couples in their circle of friends were separated or already divorced. I regarded it as completely normal that after a certain period couples lose interest in one another. The clingy goings-on at my friend's seemed a bit excessive to me. *You don't fool me,* I thought, until I saw that they were being quite honest. So I know it is possible. But rare.

There are men who are more romantic than Paul, and others I can talk to more easily. I can imagine almost anything happening between myself and other men, but cannot imagine spending my life with anyone other than Paul. We moved in together after a lovely long trip to Indonesia, where Paul's father was born. There we bought a beautiful dark woodcarving, with intertwined figures that formed a family.

With Paul I no longer saw living with a man as robbing me of my freedom. He has something that binds me to him. He is not predictable; he continually surprises me with his mental leaps and his jokes. He doesn't claim me or force me into a particular role. Perhaps I really can do it with him: be a spouse and a lover at the same time. And—why not?—a mother, too.

I know for certain that he will be a great father. Some people have children—others have a way with children. He falls into the second category. He's always known that he wants children. In my case, children was something for *later*. Now it *is* later. We walk to where we are staying and make love as if it is our first night together, tender and passionate. I am super-stitious: A child is created through love. I'm quite certain we've hit the mark.

Months later we receive a telephone call from France. Paul's father has had a stroke while on vacation. Dick is lying, his one side paralyzed, in a French hospital. We leave immediately. Dick can no longer talk, and he doesn't react to anything. For the first time since I've known Paul, I see tears in his eyes. We're afraid that Dick will die or, worse still, not recover. The whole family gathers in the small vacation house, where fear, anxiety, and excessive cheerfulness alternate with one another. It is a culture shock for this family, which has never had a strong tra-dition of intimacy. Paul's mother died young and left Dick with three small children. He was broken and had no idea how to deal with the children's grief. He took care of them, but their mother was never spoken of again. Dick met his second wife, Gwen, when the children had already left home.

Paul's stepmother had also had her fair share of misery in the past, but she was a talker with no qualms about reopening old wounds. It was, in fact, thanks to her that any kind of family ties developed. And now, through his stroke, Dick is organizing the first real family reunion. Between visits to the hospital, we talk, cry, and laugh as if our lives depend on it. For me it is the first time I have been in close proximity to such a great loss. Paul and I forget completely that we have for some time been trying to procreate. Now we make love to banish the specter of death. It helps.

Dick starts to talk again, in odd bombastic sentences: "From which official authority in this institution did you obtain this information?" And: "The circulation of air in this room is extremely pleasant." Malay words pepper his speech. He spent the first twenty years of his life in Indonesia. He was born of an Indonesian mother and a Dutch father.

Paul looks like him. He has the same attractive slim build, the same creative and independent spirit, and the same boundless curiosity. Although Dick is still lying in the hospital with his skewed Popeye mouth, he has his Walkman on and is once again enjoying his latest discovery: the music of Tom Waits, which Paul's brother brought him. We learn that the bleeding was so severe that there are many things Dick will never be able to do again. He had played a lot of tennis, and he'd intended to keep on working until the day he died. Now he'll have to put those ideas right out of his poor head.

My hands itch when I see him struggling with the strap of his watch, and I stifle my "Can I help you?" But after an interminably long period of fiddling, he does it himself. I am impressed by his patience and perseverance. How does he do it? Slowly he learns to talk again, to walk and to use both hands, although with the necessary limitations. He has chronic pain in his foot, tires quickly, and has trouble concentrating for long. Still, he continues to enjoy life as he always has. I hope Paul will get old like that, too. But without the stroke, of course.

It took more than a year, but now it has happened. I feel extremely sexy. Just as a brand-new mother goes around forcing everyone to look at the photos of her offspring, I walk around flaunting my breasts. In just a few months, they have become startlingly large and firm, and marvelously sensitive. It is as if I have acquired a sixth sense. I feel as hot as a queen bee!

I am so full of my pregnancy that I mention it to everyone who is willing to listen. In this way it also becomes more real for me. My friends Isabel, Lisa, and Natasha give me a book, *Pregnancy and Childbirth*. They have written well-meaning messages in it, saying that they definitely want to babysit and that growing up with an au pair can also be fun. They tell me I am mad for voluntarily choosing the constraints that come with having a child, especially since I haven't even reached the magical limit of thirty yet. But they also find it interesting: I am the first in our group. In exchange for the book, I allow them to see my bare breasts. Their reaction is appropriately admiring.

One of my friends, Anna, already has a child. Because she did not have a man in her life at that point, she asked me to be present at the delivery. She delivered on a birthing stool next to her bed, as I sat behind her, to support her. Between the labor pains she would drop back into my arms and I would brush her hair away from her sweat-bathed face. While she was pushing I folded myself around her, like a living armchair, and she pinched my legs until I was black and blue. When the pain shot through her, I absorbed it into my body. The great flood of release, too, I felt start up within me. I had put a mirror at her feet so that she could see what was happening. Anna was half unconscious from the effort, but I saw the little head appear and the tiny body burst from inside her. Everything was streaming—blood, amniotic fluid, tears. I was allowed to cut the umbilical cord. Her daughter was named after me. Judith is now four and also wants to marry Paul, later on.

My mother and Paul's stepmother think it's fantastic that I am pregnant. My mother already has three grandchildren from my eldest brother, but she would like to have a lot more. Every new life in the family seems to be a belated victory over the Nazis, who murdered her mother, aunts, nieces, and nephews.

The grandchildren constitute her personal compensation, but also her triumph: You don't get rid of us that easily!

Gwen has two daughters from a previous marriage, but no grandchildren yet. One of her daughters, Lois, would love to have a child, but she is living with a man who had himself sterilized when he was in his twenties. Simon was so sure he would never want children that he even managed to convince his doctor. Some people persuade others more easily than themselves. Now he's had an operation to undo the procedure, but it appears that after years of being cut off, one's seed doesn't necessarily recover. Gwen's other daughter, Irene, has Down syndrome and has also been sterilized. There was no need to convince anyone in that case.

Paul himself has another brother and a sister, but there doesn't seem to be much chance of them reproducing. His sister is a lesbian, and his brother's relationships never last long. Paul thinks it's great that his father's family name will be passed on, although I suspect Dick isn't particularly concerned; as long as we are happy. Simon and Lois react stiffly to our news. No doubt they are jealous. My younger brother is surprised—you, already?—and starts to tease me with visions of a future filled with dirty diapers and whining. In two years' time, he'll come and visit again, he says, when the child is out of diapers and starting to talk. My father has to recover from the shock before, visibly moved, he takes me in his arms. He still sees me as his little princess. My elder brother, who speaks from experience, says solemnly that having children enriches one's life. He and his wife are thrilled at the idea of having a nephew or niece, as is my younger sister.

The only place I *don't* talk about my pregnancy is at work. I have a temporary contract as an editor with a publishing house. They are considering giving me a permanent position. Perhaps they'll change their minds if they know I am expecting a child.

I am twelve weeks pregnant. I read everything I can about pregnancy and for the first time in my life I look at baby clothes. I buy a little cotton jacket with a cute lace collar and carefully put it away in the cupboard. For myself I buy a wider pair of pants, as I'm putting on weight quite rapidly. Paul often puts his hands on my growing belly in a protective way. Every so often I forget that I am pregnant, but am reminded by his glance. He looks at me differently, more intensely, curiously, and surprised.

We start to think about names. I decide, to my own surprise, that I would like our child to have a Jewish name. I had never thought that I would want to pass on something of a family heritage in this way. I didn't think I cared about tradition or genealogy. But now that I am pregnant, I feel part of a larger whole. I am going to bind the past with the future by bringing a child into the world. My mother has a family tree of the maternal side of my family. On one closely written page, all the names end with a morbid sameness in the identical place and the identical year: Auschwitz 1943. I want to breathe new life into one of the names. Paul agrees.

I look at photos of myself and Paul as babies and children to get an idea of what our child might look like. In my family, jokes are often made about the strong genes on the maternal side. You recognize family members from miles away by their round cheeks, sparkling eyes, and heavy eyebrows. When a new child is born, there is a satisfied declaration that the little one also has "the stamp." I myself am only partially blessed with the coarse dark beauty of my mother's family. I inherited my father's calm hazel eyes. Opinion is divided over whether I look more like my father or my mother. It's all the same to me: They are both good-looking. Paul has bright blue eyes, and as a child he had really blond hair, despite his father's Indonesian blood. Genetic characteristics sometimes skip a generation. Perhaps our child will look Indonesian. I would rather he or she be dark than really blond and blue-eyed. I hope our baby will have our family stamp combined with the fine facial features of Paul's family. Musical, lively, and intelligent—and healthy, of course.

After the examination the midwife says that everything feels fine. The only thing is that she can't yet hear the heart beating. That doesn't mean anything, she says, it often happens. The baby is probably lying too deep in my abdomen, out of range of the stethoscope. I had been looking forward to the first sign of life. At my insistence we agree that I will have an ultrasound in two weeks' time.

On the day before the ultrasound appointment, things start to rumble around in my belly. We are just on our way to a cultural center where my favorite Spanish author is going to be interviewed for television. I had helped set up the interview. It had been difficult for Paul to get away from work to accompany me. In front of the theater, I break out in a cold sweat. I feel as if I might faint at any moment. It feels just like the first time I had a period. I have to go home. I have to lie down. "Things are not as they should be in there," I say to Paul, pointing at myself. He takes me home, annoyed and concerned, and then leaves to do some shopping at the market.

I lie down on the bed. Then the bleeding starts. I ring the midwife. "Occasional bleeding is completely normal," she says. "It happens fairly often. Don't worry."

I try to relax. Paul should have been back ages ago. The pain becomes almost unbearable. I drag myself to the toilet and remain sitting there because I feel too weak to go back to the bedroom. Suddenly I can feel that I am losing more than blood. I hear a plopping sound under me. The cramps immediately start decreasing. I know that I have had a miscarriage, but I cannot comprehend the meaning of what has happened. All I feel is physical relief. I stand up to look, but I cannot identify an embryo in the glistening bloody mass. But it will be in there.

I have never heard or read about what others do in such a situation. Should I go and fetch some kind of equipment to see if the embryo can be seen if I move the membrane away? A little stick? A knife and fork? Or would it be better to go and bury it in the garden at once? You're not allowed just to bury a corpse in a garden; there are rules that have to be considered. But surely an embryo isn't a corpse? Perhaps I should wait for Paul to get back, so that we can do it together. But I'm annoyed with Paul for leaving me alone. Should I simply flush it away? Or take it out and throw it in the garbage? Then I can shock him with the news: "Your child is in the trash."

Keep it, I decide; perhaps it should be examined. I get a serving spoon from the kitchen, lift the wobbly mass out of the toilet bowl, and put it into a plastic container. Perhaps I should have let it cool down first, I think, as I make room in the freezer between a plastic bag full of squid and a vacuum-packed chicken, lying awkwardly on its back, with its legs up in the air. Then I rinse the serving spoon carefully and put it back in the drawer. Only then do I notice how badly my legs are shaking. I must get back to bed. Paul is still not home. I ring Isabel, but she is not in. Natasha is, though. She comes at once and holds me tight. Now at last I can cry. And drink as much wine as I like.

Paul met a friend at the supermarket, and they went to the bar together. No, perhaps it wasn't such a good idea to have stayed away for so long. In retrospect. But he couldn't have foreseen what happened, could he? I always look for psycho-logical explanations for other people's behavior. I picked up the habit at home. I explain Paul's tendency to flee—which is not new to me—by the way his mother's death was dealt with at home. Sorrow cannot be shared; you have to forget it as quickly as possible. If you pretend it isn't there, it disappears by itself. That's how he was conditioned; he can't do anything about it.

This time it does not help much to think this. I start to wonder whether it is such a good idea to share my life with a man who opts out at crucial times. There could be so many disasters to come. The older you get, the more hassles you are likely to experience. Up to now we have got along really well, but there was no skill in that, because everything has gone smoothly. But in time we will have children. What if one of them becomes seriously ill, or dies?

My mother accompanies me to the ultrasound appointment at the hospital the next day. I have decided to go ahead with it anyway, just to make sure. I can't quite believe that after such a buildup, a pregnancy can be completely over so quickly. I have to drink a lot of water beforehand, so that my bladder feels as if it is going to burst in the waiting room. When I am finally lying on the examination bed, I forget about the pressure for a moment. On the monitor I see an unmistakable embryo. It already has a human form, a head, a trunk, little arms and legs. You see! I only lost blood and mucus! I am still pregnant! My heart starts beating faster, but the doctor gives his verdict: "There is no longer any heart activity. This is a fetus about twelve weeks old. The pregnancy was therefore terminated a week or two ago. It was probably a two-egg pair of twins, and you lost the other fetal matter yesterday."

I am taken aback by the term "fetal matter," hear myself politely thanking the doctor for the information, snatch up my clothes, and run to the toilet. First pee. Then vomit. Then cry.

My mother puts her arm around me as we walk out of the hospital together. Comfortingly she says, "Well, twins would have been dreadfully awkward. You would have been so busy, you have no idea. I really wouldn't have liked to babysit twins, you know."

I remember another time she tried to comfort me, years ago. My first great love affair had just ended. I had been with a young man to whom I was so strongly attracted that even in public we could not keep our hands off one another—to the annoyance of everyone around us. We were completely absorbed in one another. Older people found him rude, but I thought he was independent, authentic, and unconventional. He did not shake hands on principle; he thought it a meaningless social convention. I would have loved to have been as left-wing as he was, but I was too frivolous for that. He left for

Nicaragua to support the revolution. I went on a world trip and had one amorous adventure after another. I reported these to him in detail in my letters, because jealousy was bourgeois and we had an open relationship. But when I got back, he had in the meantime found another great love. I hadn't expected such a radical kind of unfaithfulness. I shed streams of tears into my pizza. As my mother took a bite of hers, she said, "Well, it's for the best. He was after all a maladjusted young man."

Giving comfort is an art that few people master, no matter how good their intentions. People often think that they are comforting someone by saying, "Chin up, it could have been worse," "You'll soon forget," or "It's all for the best." But those who are looking for comfort don't want to hear that. In their minds it could not possibly have been worse; it certainly isn't for the best!

When my brother left high school, he ended up in a crisis. He did not know how to give direction to his life; he was extremely fearful of the future. He literally and figuratively froze up. At one stage it became so bad that he could hardly speak anymore. My parents, who were in the process of divorcing, did not know how to help him. My father showered him with wise advice, for which my brother had no use. It simply made his rigidity worse. One evening, in the middle of one of his well-meant monologues, my father himself burst into tears. "I so want to help you," he sobbed, "but I don't know how. I feel so sorry for you."

At this my brother also gave way to tears. In the end his feeling of powerlessness was not talked away by good advice but by being shared. This shared weeping by two men who would not normally think to shed even a single tear in someone else's presence was the first step toward my brother's recovery.

The doctor says that I should wait for the second batch of "fetal matter" to leave my body by itself. "The body has a natural inclination to get rid of dead material." He also tells me that with one's first miscarriage no examination is generally made, because usually no cause can be found. So I needn't keep the material that I still had in the freezer.

The words *fetal matter* and *material* come to me from an immense distance, as if they have nothing to do with me. Okay, then, I'll throw the material in the trash. Together with that far-too-cute cotton baby jacket, which I should never have bought in the first place. How stupid to anticipate things like that!

I take alternating hot and cold baths and ride my bike over potholes to try to get rid of the other half. I ask Paul to take me really hard, pushing in deep. I want to punish my body and give it a scare, but all remains terribly calm in my belly. I no longer have very much confidence in the natural inclinations of my body. That embryo has no plans to leave my body of its own volition. I am constantly aware of the dead life in my abdomen. I read once about a postmortem in which they found a fossilized embryo in the womb of an old woman who had walked around with it for more than half a century. I mustn't think of that. I insist that they remove it surgically, but there is no space in the hospital. We contact a friend who is a gynecologist, and it suddenly appears that an emergency admission for a curettage will in fact be possible in a week's time, on Friday the thirteenth. What does it matter? Not much more can go wrong.

The week crawls by. Then finally I am allowed to go to the medical center. In the ward my mother plays a game of Scrabble with me to pass the time. Neither of us enjoys playing games, but it offers a distraction. The first and only time I had been in the hospital before was when I was about three, and I don't remember much about it. I have never had an operation. "This is not an operation, it is a small procedure," the admitting nurse reassures me. I have to wear a pair of disposable panties and a stiff cotton hospital gown and have a neat shower cap put on my head. "For hygienic purposes," the nurse explains. I also have to take off my ring, chain, and watch. Nothing of my own is allowed to go into the operating room with me. It seems like a practice run for the anesthetic I'll soon be getting: They are already making me disappear a little. Although I am perfectly capable of walking on my own, I am taken to the operating room on a hospital bed. The anesthetist shakes my hand

and introduces himself. I am grateful to him for this human gesture in such a sterile environment.

A few more people are walking around, all in the same green clothing, just like on television, in the gory medical programs that you sometimes get drawn into by accident. I catch a glimpse of a little table with medical instruments. Will they do it with a fork on a long handle? Or with a little vacuum cleaner? I try to click my thoughts along to another channel, but they remain stubbornly hooked on the instruments.

In the meantime they prepare the drip through which the anesthesia will shortly be administered. I am not afraid of needles. As a student I participated in a research program into what happens to your blood after you take birth control pills. You had to drink sugar water and have a lot of blood taken. It paid extremely well. If you relax, you feel almost nothing. I am able to relax without any problem. I am wary of anesthetics, though. I have heard that sometimes you don't come out of them.

Back in the ward Paul looks at the drip with anxious eyes. It does me good to see that he is concerned about me. The miscarriage itself does not seem to have touched him much, although I am never sure with him. He is so self-contained that I often tease him by saying that he has no feelings at all. My mother said to me that he looked pale, that he was quite confused by it all. I hadn't noticed anything. Perhaps I am so distracted by what is happening inside me that I am not aware of what it is doing to him. I feel bruised inside, as if I've been kicked hard in the stomach, and I ask for a painkiller. When the pain begins to subside, I feel a primitive need to see what was taken out of my belly. The doctor says it's not possible. "The material has already been destroyed." Everything is gone.

I am completely empty.

Paul comes up with a theory. He tells the story of a girlfriend of his who once had an abortion and felt very bad about it afterward. "That's far more difficult than a miscarriage," he says. "With an abortion you remove a healthy child. What you lose in a miscarriage could never have become a healthy child."

Flabbergasted, I object: An abortion you have voluntarily; a miscarriage happens to you. You have the opportunity to prepare yourself to some extent for an abortion; a miscarriage takes you by surprise. You have an abortion right at the beginning of your pregnancy; we had already made it through the critical first three months.

But, in fact, I simply don't want to talk about it, not in this way. So I start to cry again.

I wish Paul would also let his tears go, or at least tell me that he's also upset about it. Otherwise how can we share the loss? It must surely be a disappointment for him, too. He was happy about the pregnancy. Otherwise he wouldn't always have kissed my bulging belly so lovingly before we went to sleep: "Hello,

hello you in there," he would say. "How are you doing? Are you nice and warm in there? We're going to have a nice sleep now; you do the same. Then you'll grow big and strong."

The day after I come back from the hospital, still unsteady from the anesthetic and all my emotions, Paul once again spends far too long at the bar after work. When he eventually arrives home in a cloud of drink and cigarettes, I explode. This is not normal! If he doesn't change, he can definitely move in at the pub. I don't want to share my life with a loser who abandons me at precisely the times I need him most. And how often does that even happen! The one time that I need his support, he has to go boozing. Would he think it normal if I went off with my friends while he lay at home bleeding? And it wasn't just a "procedure," it was also his child! In fact, it was the second child we had lost in a week. And it is the second time in a week that he's let me down in such a boorish manner! Having a child is something you do together, and so is losing a child. If he is such a weakling that he can't manage that, then he can rot in hell.

Everything damn well happens to my body. He can simply go off to the office, while I lie, emptied out, on the couch. And he doesn't even have to take a day off, although I would have if I had been him. Surely it's not too much trouble to come straight home after work? Then perhaps he could find a bottle of wine at home and open it for both of us. I don't have the strength to do that yet, but I do feel the need for a drink. Didn't he think that perhaps I might also want something? That I would have appreciated his company?

Something must be done about his cowardly behavior immediately, otherwise the relationship is over. I want him to make an appointment to see a psychiatrist within a week. Paul can't bear to think about it: If there is one thing he abhors, it is scratching around in his inner life. But he gives in, in the face of my threats.

He returns triumphant from his initial interview. He told them that he'd been sent by his girlfriend. To this the psychiatrist replied: "Then you don't have a problem, your girlfriend has the problem. Tell her to make an appointment." I capitulate. I am no match for so much misunderstanding. What can one do if even the psychiatrists are crazy? Paul is a hopeless case, but I give up my battle. I am far too tired and have nothing to gain. If I end it now, who am I going to cuddle up to at night? That evening we watch a feel-good movie together on television. The film is terribly romantic and deliciously annoying. I lie on the couch with my head on his lap, and he runs his fingers through my hair. Being there is also a form of comfort. Breaking up is always still possible later, when I feel better.

My belly obtusely continues to bulge, even though there is no longer any reason for it. "Your body still has to get over the pregnancy," says the doctor. "It takes a few weeks before your hormonal balance gets back to normal."

Paul blames my fits of crying and anger on the confused hormones. This makes me cross as well, as if it's a purely physical thing, as if I'm not supposed to be emotional about the loss of the child we were expecting to have, of the twins that died inside me.

I'm not only angry with him; I'm angry with everyone who negates or trivializes my miscarriage.

My circle of friends and family is clearly split into two camps in my mind: those with whom you know where you are and those with whom you don't. My mother is not always the most tactful of people, but through her devotion she quickly wins first prize in the former category. She pops in almost every day, and if she doesn't, then she phones to let me know she is thinking of me. Gwen, who lives farther away, sends a beautiful bouquet of flowers and a lovely card. She makes the grade, too, as do Isabel, Natasha, Lisa, and Anna, who drop in to keep me company. They bring me pastries and things to read to take my mind off what has happened.

Then there are the people you suddenly don't hear from anymore. I can't accept it from my elder brother and his wife in particular, after they'd been so enthusiastic about my pregnancy. When I start having bad dreams about it, I decide to phone them and confront them with my reproach. Bottling things up only causes them to fester. They are too close to me for that. It appears they were too scared to call, because they themselves had managed to have three children without any problems. They thought it better to leave me to myself.

One of my friends has a theory about the perverse effect of good intentions. She says most misunderstandings are the result of assumptions. People assume too much and ask too little, even though asking is the best way to find out what others need. They could have called me to say that they feel bad for me. They could have asked if I'd prefer to be left alone. Then I could have said no and told my story, because that is what I want to do, tell what happened, so that it can become more real to me.

On my first visit to the bar after I'd been in the hospital, the friends we'd arranged to meet did not say a single word about the miscarriage the whole evening. I could just as well have stayed at home by myself as sit feeling so lonely among my friends in the pub. They no doubt also assumed that I'd rather not talk about it, that i will start the conversation if I do.

The self-consciousness one feels when confronted with another's loss is not unfamiliar to me. I also find sympathizing after a death difficult: What words should you choose, what tone of voice should you use? But at least in that situation there is one phrase you can fall back on: "My condolences." There is no such standard reaction for a miscarriage, so it's natural that they should find it difficult. Nonetheless I am still disappointed. These are my friends. I expect them at least to get over their shyness and show some interest or sympathy. Not to have to ask for it myself.

You also get people who do say something but miss the mark entirely. "It happens often. Every fourth pregnancy ends in a miscarriage," one told me. "Better luck next time!" another said comfortingly, as if I'd just lost a game of checkers.

Paul thinks I'm being oversensitive. "If they say nothing, you get upset, and if they do say something, it's also wrong." Perhaps so. Perhaps I'm angry about the miscarriage, and it's coming out in anger about the inability of those around me to comfort me. But still . . . all they have to do is ask: "How are you doing?" And then actually wait for the answer instead of nervously moving just a little too quickly to another subject.

Women generally wait three months before they tell anyone about their pregnancy, because the chance of a miscarriage is greatest up to that point. Then if something goes wrong, no one needs to know. As if your world isn't turned upside down twice, first by the pregnancy and then by the miscarriage. As if it is something you should be ashamed of. As if it shows that you yourself have failed somehow. Surely I am more than just a womb, damn it!

It seems as if only people who have had a similar experience themselves are able to understand. Isabel's brother, for example. He's a psychologist and now has two healthy children. His wife lost their first child much later in her pregnancy. "It was the worst thing that has ever happened to us," he told me earnestly. "The child was so full of life—in her belly, in our thoughts, in our plans for the future. It took a long time for us to get over the loss. Only after we'd had another child could we conclude the grieving process." The somewhat solemn term *grieving process,* in particular, stays in my mind. It shows acknowledgment.

When someone dies, the funeral is a form of mourning that makes it possible for the relatives to share their grief. You can all take your leave of the body together and afterward share memories of the deceased. But no one has any memories of our child. To others, it didn't even exist yet. It existed only in my belly and in my head.

With a miscarriage there are no rituals, there is no funeral. With a miscarriage there is nothing, absolutely nothing, except for the unwritten law that you bear your loss in silence.

CHAPTER TWO

FROM THE DESIRE FOR A CHILD TO A NIGHTMARE,

or

The Hunt for Tattoos and a Zest for Life

Instead of having twins I get a new job. At the moment I should have been giving birth, the interview is held. As a result of technical problems, my train to the city is delayed. As I get off the train, I catch my pantyhose on the handle of my bag and immediately there is a huge run. I jump into a taxi and ask the driver to stop quickly at a shop so that I can run in to buy a new pair. I put them on in the back of the car, while the driver watches me very closely in his rearview mirror. I have dressed nicely and made myself up; I look good. But a real woman I will never be: Pantyhose are too subtle for me. I pull so hard that the new pair also succumbs under my impatient hands. There's nothing more to be done.

I arrive a quarter of an hour late and meet an irritated interviewing panel. I lift my leg up in the air so that my run pantyhose show while I take the other pair out of my bag. The pantyhose are the problem; it is not my fault that I am so late. The panel laughs, and from that moment on the conversation becomes very relaxed and pleasant.

A few days later I hear that they want me, in part, because of my flair and my talent for getting out of a tight corner. Now

Paul and I both have the type of job we had hoped for: he as a journalist with a renowned daily newspaper and I as an editor with a publisher in the city. We open a bottle of wine and drink to the future.

I'm on my way back from the supermarket with my sister, plastic bags hanging from our hands. We have been shopping together. She is noticeably quiet. Just before we say goodbye, she says, "I have something to tell you. I am pregnant." Four months already. Everyone knows, except me. She is clearly nervous now that she has finally had the courage to tell me. My little sister is having a baby before me. That is against the natural order of things! My brother has four children now. But he is older, though not much. His wife got pregnant with the fourth one around the time I had my miscarriage.

I'm a bit insulted that no one in the family had the courage to tell me. I am apparently regarded as someone who must be spared this type of news. But I am more shocked than jealous. As far as I am concerned, I have put my miscarriage completely behind me. The cliché that time heals all seems to be true. Just over a year ago, I still got angry about unfeeling remarks like, "Bad luck, better luck next time." Now I think the same thing myself.

Things are going well between Paul and I again. I no longer feel like sending him to a psychiatrist; we'd rather use our free time to do fun things. We take a dancing class, go out, and enjoy nice vacations together. My work takes up so much of my time that I hardly ever even think about children anymore. I am good at this job; it satisfies me. It is full of variety, and it is exciting. I attend book fairs in Africa, Asia, and Latin America, and I enjoy the contact with publishers and writers from all over the world. I am brimming with ambition and impatience. Once I have gained enough experience in this field, I want to become a publisher with a literary publishing house. It can't come quickly enough for me.

I am unable to imagine very clearly what place children would have in this vision of the future. Most publishers are men and married to their jobs. They are either yuppies or traditional: If they already have children, they also have a wife at home looking after them. Female publishers don't have children, with the odd exception.

Do I want to become such an exception? I am always most aware of what I do not want. I do not want to become a stressed-out career woman with only quality—not quantity— time for my children. I certainly do not want to become a mother hen who never lets her children out of her sight and is herself hardly able to talk anything but baby language. But what I want least of all is to wait too long to have children.

My parents were young, energetic, and active. They compensated for their lack of communication with a busy social life. With four children on the backseat, they took long trips through Europe, in a convoy with other families or single uncles or aunts. There were always other children to play with. At home we often had guests, parties, and sleepovers. Provided you didn't make too much noise or whine, you could stay up well into the night without anyone thinking of sending you to bed. I'd like to take having children in my stride, as a natural part of my life, without having to give up working and seeing friends, partying, and traveling. You probably have to be young and you certainly have to be flexible for that, though. At thirty-one I am already starting to wonder whether I can, in fact, fit kids into my life. One more sign that I should not hesitate any longer. At my age my mother already had four children, and now even my youngest sister is pregnant. And so with a theatrical gesture, I throw my diaphragm, which since the miscarriage has had a place of honor next to my bed, into the garbage.

I'm still not pregnant. I keep track of the fertile periods in my cycle and then call Paul: "Come, we're going to make another baby!" We try absolutely everything to get a positive result. If I see a falling star, I don't ever have to think about my wish. A friend gives me a chain with a little stone on it that I have to wear directly against my skin for optimal effect. The added advantage of this is that I can hide it under my clothing. The same friend tells me that her sister became pregnant after using a Chinese fertility-promoting tea.

In a reckless mood I walk into a little shop full of powders and herbs to ask whether they sell such a tea. I make sure I wait until there are no other people in the shop. The Chinese man behind the counter does not understand what I mean. I try to explain, already regretting my decision. The man calls his companion, who has a better command of the language. In the meantime new customers are coming into the shop. With red cheeks I once more whisper what I have come for and make gestures with my hands: drink, big belly. General confusion. In the end I run out of the shop. I am sure I hear them laughing inside.

On the bedside table, where my diaphragm used to lie, an African fertility doll made of colored beads now stands and grins encouragingly. Next to it is an amulet from the same continent that has already proved its efficacy several times for others. It should actually also be on a chain around my neck, but that would make things a bit overcrowded. So instead I roll it through my fingers like a rosary at night before I go to bed.

I read once that the chances are best when the man comes first and the woman shortly thereafter. The greedy womb then sucks the sperm in with its orgasmic movements and sends them up the fallopian tubes. But sometimes the reports contradict one another. According to one, the man should ejaculate at least a day before, so that the sperm—new and now better!—can head energetically toward their goal. Another holds that a few days of abstinence improves the quality of the sperm. When the little guys are finally released after a few days of lonely confinement, you can't hold them back! They don't know at that stage that they may well be heading for further imprisonment in another body.

To make sure that after all these precautions the semen does not head in the wrong direction by mistake, after we make love I lie motionless on my back with my legs in the air for minutes. I think of the words of a friend: "There is no rest for your fanny. Is it surprising that a child can't take root in you?" She should see me. Sometimes I even stand on my head so that the sperm can run along a straight line to their final destination.

It's that time of the month again. The day before I start menstruating, I invariably have a splitting headache, I am shaky, and I am unsure about everything. It has always been that way. Before I started keeping track of my cycle, I took the existential angst very seriously. I would decide that I was making a mess of my life, that I could do nothing, and that I was worth nothing. The following day I would breathe a sigh of relief when I discovered the cause of my depressive state of mind.

I was thirteen when I started my periods, and I had been looking forward to them. Other girls in my class had already started, and they had a special status that I envied. They were women. But once I had begun, I no longer understood why I had been so eager.

The first time, I was literally floored. It was during a summer holiday in France, and the staff in the shop in which I fainted immediately called an ambulance. If my mother had not interfered, they would have taken me off to the hospital.

I had never actually fainted before—it was an extraordinary feeling. First the blood leaves your head, then you get cold and your legs get weak, and the next moment you are gone. You only notice this when you come around again and find yourself lying on the ground. From far away you can hear snatches of sound, and it slowly dawns on you that they are voices saying, "Goodness, but she is pale." Even later you realize that they are talking about you. That is the moment that you are fully conscious again.

The first year, this happened to me on a regular basis, a number of times during class. It broke the routine of the school day, and one of my classmates was allowed to take me home. But it was not unadulterated pleasure, because the fainting spell was followed by severe stomach cramps. Later I learned to suppress these by using strong painkillers. There was a whole art to getting the pink bombs down your throat.

When I went on the pill at sixteen, my menstruation problems disappeared. But the pill brought on other discomforts. It made me put on weight, and I forgot to take it. The desperate remedy of the morning-after pill made me really sick. After using the pill for ten years, I was so fed up that I chose the hassle of condoms or a diaphragm. All a waste of time, it now appeared. All the menstruation problems, the hordes of hormones in your body, the efforts to prevent conception. All from the ridiculous fear of becoming pregnant, when there was no more reliable contraceptive than my own body!

While deep-sea diving in Honduras, I saw a beautiful dolphin on someone's shoulder. Since then I have been fantasizing about a tattoo and know this has something to do with my inability to get pregnant. I want something irreversible, something I myself can put on my body at the time I choose. And that I can be certain will stay there.

One day after a tedious business meeting, I walk into a tattoo parlor. Fascinated, I look at all the photos and drawings on the wall. It looks like an anthropological museum—images of tattooed skin are everywhere. In the area next door I hear a drilling sound, like at the dentist. I peer around the corner: A heart that has faded on an upper arm is being colored bright red again. The owner of the heart does not flinch.

35

A heavily tattooed man asks if he can help me. He is wearing a pair of shorts, and his upper body is bare. There is not a spot on his skin that is not colored. I feel naked in my coat and skirt with so much uncovered skin everywhere: my arms, my legs, my throat, completely bare. I ask whether he does dolphins, which suddenly seems like a childish request. But he takes out a file full of dolphins. Big dolphins, small dolphins, dolphins in pairs jumping over one another, dolphins jumping through a ring, dolphins leaping out of the sea. I ask whether I may take a sample home, so I can show it to my boyfriend and he can think about it, too.

The tattooed man reacts indignantly: "No, of course you can't. Are you mad? These are unique designs. We can't just hand them out." I'm still not sure, but my desire to do something definite overcomes my hesitation. I select a dolphin leaping out of the sea. I like dolphins because they are mobile, sensuous, supple, strong, and intelligent; they even seem to have a sense of humor. They live in the sea, but manage at the same time through their own power to free themselves from it, to leap into the air and then to dive back joyously into their own element. I am also in my element in the sea. There I feel myself to be in harmony with my environment; there I feel alive. I enjoy nothing more than diving into the surf and letting myself be carried along by the power of the waves. The idea of carrying something of that power with me, on my own shoulder, appeals to me.

I am quite sure that the tattoo has to go on my shoulder. However, the shoulder appears to be a broad concept. When I have to indicate exactly where I want the dolphin, I am at a loss. Relieved, I leave it to the expert, who immediately works out the correct position. Then comes the choice of colors. Red and black are my favorites.

The tattooed giant blusters: "Red and black? A dolphin is blue or gray, or blue-gray, or blue-green, but not red and black!" There is some truth in what he says. I meekly select a blue-green, although it is not my color at all. I do not have a single turquoise piece of clothing, but I wisely hold my tongue about that. It would be like saying to an artist: "Your painting does not match the color of my bedroom suite." I actually want to go home, but it is too late. Very soon I am sitting with the top of my body exposed next to the guy with the faded heart. The pain isn't too bad. It is almost pleasant. Afterward a bandage is put over it.

Paul takes the bandage off that evening and holds a hand mirror up so I can see the tattoo reflected in the larger mirror. We are as excited as if it were the unveiling of a monument we had erected. The dolphin is lovely—not too large, not too small, not too coarse, but fine and elegant. The sea is the only thing I don't like. It is almost the same color as the dolphin, and so it looks like an extension of the animal. As if the waves are pulling the dolphin down by its tail. The animal wants to get free of the sea but cannot. The force of gravity from the sea is stronger than the upward leap of the dolphin. I thought that I would feel strong and confident with this tattoo, but the opposite is true. I just had to do something irreversible, but I had no idea what I was doing. I didn't think carefully enough about exactly how I wanted it. I acted far too impulsively. Perhaps I was not born for irrevocable deeds.

We go to our family doctor for advice. Perhaps there is a demonstrable reason why I am not getting pregnant. "So you have a desire for a child?" the doctor asks sympathetically. We answer in the affirmative, although we have never thought about it in those terms. We have to tell him how often we have sexual relations. He advises us to keep a systematic record of when I am in my fertile cycle, using the temperature method. He gives us a diagram on which we can plot a fertility curve with little crosses so that we can see exactly when ovulation occurs. That is the pivotal moment. In the days just before, during, and after this, there is the greatest chance of success. From now on we mustn't let those days pass unused. Making love at the right time, that is the secret. In addition he gives us a pamphlet, *If Getting Pregnant Is Difficult,* to read at home. And we have to have a whole series of fertility tests at the hospital.

I stuff the pamphlet and the reference to the hospital deep into my bag. On the way home deathly weariness comes over me and stays with me for days. It is almost a week before I can bring myself to fish the pamphlet out of my bag and phone the hospital for an appointment. Up to now we simply wanted a baby, but since the visit to the doctor we have a Desire for a Child. It sounds like a disease that might well be incurable.

The foundations of our house are sinking badly. Leaks develop under the house. Another few years and it will have to be pulled down. From the time we find out about this, we do nothing further about it, since the deterioration can't be stopped. You can see it in the walls, which slowly but surely are starting to show signs of cracks. You can also smell it: When you come home, you're greeted by the damp musty smell. Recently I discovered mold under our mattress.

In the meantime, pregnancies and births are occurring all around us. Every birth announcement, not to mention visits to the new mothers, confronts me with our own inadequacy. I feel like putting a sticker on the front door that says: NO BIRTH ANNOUNCEMENTS PLEASE.

You recognize them at once from the small size and the stamp with a stork on it; sometimes the envelope is also a pale pastel color. I often leave envelopes like these unopened. I certainly can't afford to feel the tears burning behind my eyes all day long at work. Unwillingly I eventually tear the envelope open and glance at the beautiful illustration or baby photo. Then I open up the card and read the text very quickly. It rarely says anything original. On the left appears the archaic warning, "Please phone to arrange a visit." As if in this country, in this day and age, anyone would even think of arriving unannounced to visit someone, let alone someone who has just had a baby. As if we are all just dying to share in that initial joy. On the right appears the triumphant proclamation: "We are proud to announce the birth of our child." As if they have earned it! The braggarts. It's just dumb luck!

I have to force myself to exhibit the enthusiasm you are obliged to show in this situation. If I can get away with sending a card, I do so. If I have to go and visit the new mother, I put it off as long as possible, until the first rose-colored clouds have cleared.

But the babies aren't the worst. I have more trouble with the presence of a pregnant belly than with a baby. Babies are innocent; they are simply there. But pregnant bellies are provocative, offensive. Pregnant bellies confront you with a promise that in your case has not been fulfilled. Their fullness reflects your emptiness. Their pride, your failure. When you visit a new mother you always meet pregnant women, friends from prenatal classes who will be giving birth soon. And if they are not pregnant, then they have been, or they know someone who is.

The most annoying thing about visits to new mothers is the monotonous chatter about pregnancy and delivery. I cannot join in these conversations, because my experience in this area is inappropriate for such happy gatherings. I am a sheep that has fallen into the ditch and scrambled out on the wrong side from the rest of the flock. The divide appears far deeper than I had ever imagined.

So I stand and watch the rest of the herd happily cavorting around from a distance. I try with all my might to make myself invisible. But there is always an interested mother-in-law or sister who tries to get me involved by asking whether I also have any children or am going to be having any. I have tried a variety of answers, but there is no correct answer when the situation is so painful that I am unable to say anything good about it. I could say no and start talking about something else. Sometimes it works, but at other times it's just not enough and they want to know all the ins and outs. I could say that I'd like to have children but that it isn't happening very easily in our case. I know exactly the compassionate look that I get then. I hate that look. Recently I tried saying laughingly: "No, we're not very good at making children." A man who heard this remark asked me whether he should come over and demonstrate. Jewish jokes aren't funny either, when they are told by non-Jews.

It begins to dawn on me that there is something fundamentally wrong with our ability to propagate. It is a completely debilitating realization. I am used to having things more or less under control. If I really want something, I go for it heart and soul, and generally I am successful.

Getting my driver's license is one of the things that gave me a huge amount of trouble. I had a recurring nightmare in which I was sitting alone in the backseat of a moving car. I could not get to the steering wheel, and the car was thundering at full speed down the highway. So getting my driver's license had more than merely a practical significance for me. It symbolized the control I wanted to be able to exercise over my own life. I had innumerable driving lessons, but failed the test time and again. I used to get furious about it. The biggest idiots were sitting behind steering wheels. If they could do it, I must be able to as well. I kept at it until I had that license in my hand.

Now I am getting worked up about the fact that the biggest bunglers have children at the drop of a hat, while we, a pair of batty intellectuals, are taking measurements and keeping graphs in bed. But this time my fury doesn't help me one little bit; this is not something I can beat with perseverance. I want something that I'm apparently not going to get. And it is not just anything. It's a question of propagation, the essence of life, life itself. To think that I got into such a state about something as trivial as driving—if I could go back, I'd happily trade my driver's license for a successful pregnancy. I would like to offer a sacrifice, but I have no God before whom I can do so. People who believe in God draw comfort from Him in difficult times; He gives them hope and trust, two things I could really use at this moment. And if things still don't work out, God helps you find the necessary resignation.

My father does have a God. Over the years his religious experience has expanded. To him, reincarnation is an obvious given. He talks about a previous life as he would about a previous house. Suffering has meaning for him. By suffering, a person can grow. He is in contact with the divine in all sorts of ways. His current lover is a medium; she receives and passes on messages from above. Both do healing massages, through which they pass positive energy on to others. When we were small, he just went to church like everyone else. My mother never came along. All her life she had had a strong aversion to anything vaguely religious. Only much later did she begin to attend a liberal synagogue on Jewish feast days, but that had more to do with a feeling of solidarity than with religion.

For a long time my father continued to pray before meals. "Thank you, Lord, for this delicious food, amen," he would mumble almost incomprehensibly. But my mother, who was not particularly happy in her role as housewife, had good ears and would say sharply: "You should thank me, I'm the one that did the goddamn cooking!"

We children were allowed to choose for ourselves. As in many other cases, my mother's influence proved to be dominant. I went to church on the odd occasion, because I liked the singing and the stories, and to please my father. But I only prayed if I had lost something or if I really wanted something very badly.

It is now four years since we first thought that we would like to have a child. Friends who had not even considered it a few years ago are now all getting pregnant. I don't begrudge them this, but I am jealous of them—mostly of the way their pregnancies occur as a matter of course. It is so normal for them that they even feel entitled to complain: They are troubled by morning sickness, are tired, or are concerned.

I am also jealous of ambitious women who do not want children and enthusiastically dedicate themselves to their work. They're not worried whether they are fertile or not. The world seems full of enviable women: pregnant women and career women. I find myself in the no man's land in between. Why do I have such a need to be pregnant? Life certainly has more to offer than runny noses and dirty diapers. I simply backed the wrong horse. I wish that I knew there was absolutely no hope. Then I could go back to where I was before this stupid desire for a child started to affect our life.

But now we have to investigate. While the examination is at the hospital around the corner, the end is not yet in sight. How much longer? Will Paul—who does not cope well with problems—be able to stand it? Or will I suddenly hear that he is going to leave me because—yes, sorry—he has fallen in love with someone else? An uncomplicated, happy girl who does not spend days in a funk after receiving a birth announcement or visiting a new mother. That is a third category of enviable women, and the most threatening: available, fertile women; possible objectives for Paul's desire to procreate. I observe him with sharp eyes and grow to dislike myself even more. That's not how I want to be: so depressed, petty, jealous, spunkless, and full of self-pity. *Frustrated woman in her thirties seeks zest for life.* But where? How?

Perhaps I should cut myself off from everything related to pregnancy and birth. Concentrate solely on my work, over which I do have control. Only associate with people who quite definitely do not want children. Men, preferably. Throw myself into going out. Avoid babies and children and never again visit a new mother. That is one of Paul's tips, and he lives according to this creed: Don't do anything that you don't want to do. But this might cost me my relationships with friends and family. That would be a high price.

I realize it is simply not feasible to avoid half the population. You bump into them all over the place. With their pregnant bodies, they block the aisles in the supermarket. With their baby carriages, they take up the whole sidewalk. Or they come toward you singing, with a gorgeous little child in the baby stroller. They also keep popping up at parties: the women who prefer to drink sparkling mineral water or oh so nonchalantly bring their babies along and have to feed them in between. Then you have to tenderly watch the greedy guzzling at the provocatively bulging breast.

Even at work you are not safe: Colleagues unceremoniously begin to coo when they hear the word *baby* or come to show off their new acquisitions. Fortunately you can hide behind your computer at work. But you can't get away from your own friends and family. You can hardly have nothing further to do with them because they have become pregnant and you haven't.

This is why I didn't say no to visiting a glowing Joyce, who until recently was still in my camp. She had also been unable to get pregnant. In solidarity we groused together about all our boring friends who were no longer any fun since they had begun a family. Now our ways have also parted. The hormones of pregnancy seem to have destroyed all her memories of more difficult times. She has already heard the heart beating. It was a very special moment, she tells me enthusiastically.

"Yes, I can imagine." I try to make it sound like I mean it. My voice sounds harsh, I clutch the bar stool, the conversation dies. It isn't going well. I mustn't withdraw into myself. I mustn't listen to the silence in my own womb. I must say something about it. Perhaps then things will go a bit better.

"I am jealous of you," I start and am immediately sorry for my outpouring. Because now I have to continue—but I am not yet able to find the right tone to bridge the new gap between us. It comes out far more heavily than I had intended. I embarrass her. I spoil the mood.

That evening I cry myself to sleep. I dream I am lying in a double bed together with Paul and Joyce. Joyce is lying in the middle, Paul pressed close up against her and half over her. I am nearly dying of jealousy and walk out of the room to use the toilet. I hear them giggling and feel excluded. When I return and Paul gets up to use the bathroom, I see his erection. I decide to be open and tell Joyce that I am jealous and would like to lie in the middle now. She says that she values my honesty enormously, but I can hear from her voice that she is, in fact, only interested in Paul. At that moment, Paul comes back and makes a snide remark about this honesty of mine. I am deeply hurt and realize that he would like me to disappear so that he can have his way with Joyce. I say that I could leave, but that he must realize that it will be for good. He says he thinks that is an excellent idea.

47

I cry out, bewildered: "You don't mean that!"

"Oh yes, I do," he says, icily. I run out of the bedroom. He locks the door after me.

I am standing naked in the passage. Crying—still or again?—I wake up. Paul pulls me against him, strokes my back soothingly, and says comfortingly: "Shhhh, my love, it will all be okay."

CHAPTER THREE

MARRIAGE AND HOME,

or

How I Bury Myself Alive in a Provincial Town

Paul has to come in a little container. He's allowed to do it at home, but then he has to get the semen to the hospital as quickly as possible, and it must be kept at body temperature. He cuddles the little plastic container against his chest like a premature kitten. He feels embarrassed when he hands it over. It looks so little when it is in a transparent container like that. Perhaps other men deliver more. But it is received routinely, and to his relief no one holds it up to the light with a scornful smile. The result is available very quickly. There are more than enough spermatozoids and there is nothing unusual about their quality or mobility. Paul takes a breath, relieved. I set my teeth. It is a lot less simple for women. There are numerous possible causes. And far from all of them are demonstrable.

First I undergo an internal examination. I have no problem with that; I've had so many already. My uterus looks great and feels normal, the gynecologist assures me. That's good to hear. Imagine if he had said: "Ma'am, your uterus doesn't look too good!" I'd rather not hear things like that. Vanity runs deep.

This is followed by the "sperm life test." For that we have to sleep with one another at a time determined by the doctors. A day later they check whether the sperm are alive in the lining of the uterus, because some women seem to eliminate their partner's seed as soon as it enters them. I hope this won't be the case with me. I don't dare wash that morning in case I destroy the evidence. When I open my legs for the doctor, the intimate smell of our togetherness wafts up, right into the gynecologist's nose. Would he find it an exciting smell, or an unpleasant one? Or does a gynecologist become immune to body odors? He doesn't move a muscle. Thank goodness it appears from the sperm life test that there is nothing wrong with our chemical interaction.

Next comes what is for the moment the last and most unpleasant test: A contrast fluid is injected into my uterus and Fallopian tubes to make them visible on the screen in order to determine whether there are any blockages in the Fallopian tubes. I am warned that this test can be painful because of the pressure the fluid may exercise on the tubes. They do not exaggerate. It feels as if I am being blown up like a balloon from inside. I am stretched further and further until I indicate that I am about to burst. Fortunately the pressing pain dissipates as soon as the injection of the fluid is stopped. I watch the screen throughout the examination, but the meaning of the images is not clear to me. Afterward I feel dizzy and sick. It is just as well Paul is there to hear the results: My left Fallopian tube is completely clear, the right one is not. That halves the chances of pregnancy, and so it's not so surprising that it is taking so long. At the same time, despite its unfortunate ending, my previous pregnancy—which was three years ago now—shows that I am not infertile. There is, therefore, no reason to lose hope. I must simply be more patient, perhaps not even for very much longer. According to the doctor it regularly happens that after going through this test a woman gets pregnant within three months.

We do all the things that thirtysomethings do. It is worryingly predictable and at the same time all new and exciting for us. We are going to get married and buy a house. I used to think that this kind of thing was reserved for middle-class frumps. Now I no longer think that narrow-mindedness and frumpishness are related to marital status or accommodation. You find these characteristics in all sections of the population and no doubt also in alternative circles. Previously I regarded marriage as a repressive institution, invented to curtail individual freedom. In essence I still believe this, but living together falls into the same category, and we have been doing that for years. And you have to live somewhere, whether you pay rent or a mortgage.

Through my relationship with Paul, I have come to regard freedom and independence in a different way. Absolute freedom is worthless, because it is synonymous with indifference. I still think that Paul is the nicest person around and the one with whom I would most like to share my life. We've been a couple a long time, so why not marry? Marriage is a public declaration of love to the person you want to be with. It is also an excuse for a big celebration. We haven't given a party for ages. We have been together for ten years now, and we want to celebrate this on a large scale. Precisely because no one expects it of us, we think marrying will be a nice way of doing so. And some people become pregnant by getting married.

The wedding day is not yet in sight, but the test is unmistakably positive. I run to Paul with it so that he can see with his own eyes. One blue dot means you are not pregnant, two blue dots mean you are, I explain to him. He does not trust my explanation and reads the directions himself before he acknowledges that according to this test I am, indeed, pregnant. But he keeps his level-headed approach: wait and see how things develop.

I, however, am elated. The most important threshold has been crossed: The pregnancy is a fact. We have been trying for so long, and now we have succeeded. How things develop will obviously become clear only with time. But I don't want to spoil my mood with the concern that something might go wrong. This time I won't have a worry-free pregnancy, but that doesn't mean I can't at least be glad that I am pregnant. I won't buy any baby clothes this time, nor think about names, nor fantasize about what the child might look like and what it will feel like to hold it in my arms. I will be expecting without expecting anything. It sounds like an impossible contradiction.

The house we want to buy has a garden, with the sea and the dunes nearby—much nicer for children than the city. It is late-nineteenth century, with a large balcony with French doors, glass in lead frames, a lot of original woodwork, and orna-mental work on the ceiling. Everything is larger and more spacious and nicer than our current home. It smells like wood and happiness.

We worry whether it is far too large. But everyone says that too much space is never a problem. As we walk through, we try to imagine the house arranged to suit us. I hear myself say to Paul: "That would make a nice nursery." I quickly cor-rect myself: "Or study." Paul laughs and runs his hand gently over my belly.

Anna and her daughter come for dinner. Usually Anna brings a nice bottle of wine with her. This time she has a plant. Just as I am about to put it down, she says: "It is called luck-in-the-bedroom." I startle on hearing the name and look at the plant more carefully. It is small and tender. Under normal circumstances it would last little more than a week or two under my loveless care. Now I will give it a place of honor in our home and look after it carefully. It is almost a test of competency. If it stays alive, the child in my abdomen will also live.

In view of my "history" I am allowed to have an ultrasound after six weeks. It seems that they should be able to register heart activity in the womb as early as that. Nervously I go to the hospital, where, after all the tests, I am becoming a regular. I am booked in the gynecological section and am allowed to go straight through to the ultrasound room. As I lie on the familiar examination bed with my legs apart, I wonder what someone who does ultrasounds for a living is called. Definitely not an ultrasounder. But then what? I don't have the courage to ask. The last thing I want is to distract the ultrasounder, or whatever she is called. She is assiduously searching for an embryo in my womb. It takes an awfully long time. Could she be inexperienced? It seems impossible to me to get lost in a uterus. "Ultrasounder"—it would look rather odd on a business card, wouldn't it? Or if you have to introduce yourself: "How do you do? I am the ultrasounder from Our Lady Hospital." Still she says nothing. Could something be wrong?

"Are you sure you are pregnant?" she eventually asks.

"The test was positive," I say. "The tests are reliable, aren't they?"

She nods and once again moves the device from left to right and back again. The thing is much like a vibrator, but arouses absolutely no lustful feelings.

"Well, the lining of the uterus is thicker than normal," says the ultrasounder. "That indicates pregnancy activity. But I can't find the embryo. Perhaps the pregnancy started later than you think and it is simply not yet visible." I can hardly imagine this being possible. For a long time now, we haven't left anything to chance.

She gives me a folder with her notes in it to give to the gynecologist, with whom I have an appointment after this. In the waiting room I read her notes. It is my file, after all. I nonetheless feel as if I'm doing something I shouldn't. My eyes are caught by the phrase "extra-uterine gravidity" with a question mark behind it. I took Latin at school. My heart turns over: She suspects that I have an ectopic pregnancy.

The doctor looks at the photos, and I have to undergo another internal examination. Once again everything feels absolutely normal and seems fine. He says nothing else, and I don't ask anything either, partly so that it is not obvious I have read the notes and partly from nerves. He once again refers me to the laboratory to have some blood taken.

When I phone for the results the following day, the doctor fires off a rapid monologue. Nothing can yet be said with certainty, but it looks as if we might be dealing with a pregnancy that is not going to develop properly. The fetus might be stuck in my right Fallopian tube. That is the one that is partially blocked anyway. The problem is that an ectopic pregnancy can seldom be picked up properly in an ultrasound. They don't want to operate unnecessarily. There is a good chance that the fetus may be eliminated or broken down by the body itself. So the best would be to wait another week and see, in the hope that this happens, so that surgical intervention is not necessary. But if I have severe abdominal pains or bleeding, I must contact the hospital immediately.

The doctor hangs up, after first wishing me an enjoyable day. What was it he actually said? Do I really have an ectopic pregnancy? I decide to take only the words "nothing can yet be said with certainty" seriously and go on with my work as if nothing is wrong. I am damn well not going to let it get me down.

Only that evening at home, when I have to repeat his words to Paul, does it begin to dawn on me: We can forget about this pregnancy, and if I am unfortunate, I will have to have an operation as well. I am starting to think that I must have been a child murderer in a previous life.

It is a déjà vu experience: We have to wait a week, even though we already know that things are not right at all. Waiting is terrible, especially when you know that there is no way the outcome can be positive. But in this case I don't feel inclined to insist on being admitted to the hospital, because I am hoping an operation won't be necessary.

Thank heavens I am extremely busy at work, and every now and again I manage to think of something else. After a few days I have a pain in my abdomen.

In the waiting room at the hospital, I run into a highly pregnant Maria. Paul went to bed with her during the initial stages of our relationship, before we had worked out a code of conduct for intimate relations with third parties. Before I started going out with Paul, I had had a number of boyfriends and was never monogamous. I wanted to get as much as I could out of life. But Paul was a serial monogamist. So he came to me, conscious of his guilt, and fell pathetically to his knees in front of me as he confessed: "I have strayed."

I had never used or heard the expression in relation to myself. I viewed it as something for long-married couples and felt like bursting into laughter, but at the same time I felt a sharp pang of jealousy. I had never been so much in love and naturally assumed it was mutual. Paul had asked officially if I wanted to go out with him, also an oddly old-fashioned concept. At first I thought he was using the expression ironically, and when it appeared that this was not the case, I felt strangely moved. He had ended his previous relationship for me. Now, in retrospect, I was sorry for giving myself uncondi-

tionally to him. Perhaps the shine was already off it for him,
now that the conquest had been made. Except that I had
thought it went further than that with us. Perhaps I was wrong.
Perhaps I was already going to be traded in.

"Do you love her?" I asked anxiously. No, he didn't love her,
he loved me. That was a relief. On the other hand, my pride
was wounded. I thought that I was the frivolous party in mat-
ters of love. This turnaround wasn't to my liking at all, but I
wasn't going to admit it and said matter-of-factly: "I don't have
a problem with you going to bed with others, provided you
don't object if I do the same." He shuddered visibly at the
thought and cried from the bottom of his heart: "No, please
no!" The despair in his voice amused me. Apparently we were
well matched.

A month later something happened that once again
aroused my jealousy to the extreme. Maria thought that she
was pregnant by Paul. If this was the case, she wanted to keep
it, because she wanted to have a child, preferably with a partner, but if need be without one. Paul didn't know what to think
about it. He was four years older than me, and he did want children, although not necessarily there and then. I was twenty-
two and nowhere near ready for children. But if Maria was to
have his child, I would undoubtedly lose Paul. It would create a
bond between them that I would have no part of. Just thinking
about it gave me a stomachache. To her disappointment and
my relief, she eventually turned out not to be pregnant. After

that, Paul and I promised to be faithful to one another. To avoid jealousy and other misery.

Now it is ten years later, and Maria has finally achieved this fiercely desired status. She is pregnant with twins. However the examinations have indicated that something is not right. The children might be slow in their growth or their development. It is also possible that nothing will be wrong. She is finding the uncertainty difficult to cope with. The man by whom she is pregnant has opted out. As a result of circumstances and all the worries and discomfort of her pregnancy, she is unable to work. My initial envy at the sight of her belly ebbs away.

I tell her about my situation: first a miscarriage of twins and now an ectopic pregnancy. But still with Paul, good job, nice house. We catch up within a few minutes, like old friends who get the picture from a single word. When my name is called, we embrace one another and wish one another all the best. A strange association through circumstance. We not only shared the same man, but we are also both concerned about what is happening inside our bodies.

Naturally men also can have concerns about their baby-making abilities, but their concerns are located at another, less intrinsic level. Their physical involvement comprises a release of sperm. After that, it is literally finished. Their moods are not determined by hormones in the service of reproduction. They experience no menstrual pain, no pregnancy complaints, no delivery pains. They can direct all their time and energy to things outside themselves. Only when they are ill do their bodies get in the way.

Women have no less chance of getting sick than men. However, for around five days every month—some sixty days a year—they also have their period. And that continues for at least thirty years, which works out to eighteen hundred days— a total of five years! If you have two or three children, you can add another two years or so of possible pregnancy-related problems. Women are thus distracted for easily seven years of their lives by their own bodies. And this is in the ideal situation where everything goes smoothly. "You get so much in return," say those in the know.

The gynecologist thinks that the pain in my abdomen is probably the result of the production of pregnancy hormones, because the pain is on the left and according to him the pregnancy is on the right. So he does not find it worrying.

A few days later, on the way to the station, I double over as a result of a sudden stabbing on the left side of my lower abdomen. I get back home as quickly as I am able and phone the hospital. I must come in immediately, they say. I call for a taxi, but none are available for at least half an hour. Under normal circumstances it would take me five minutes to get there by bike. How long it takes me this time, I have no idea. I cannot sit on the saddle, so I cycle bent forward. When I arrive at the hospital, I am clearly in a bad state, because within the shortest possible time I am lying in a bed. Or perhaps it only seems like this; I have no concept of time, I am half drugged by the pain. Sometimes I am aware of where I am. Someone asks whether there is anyone they should notify, and I remember Paul's existence. The number is dialed for me, and thank goodness he realizes he must come at once, even though it will probably be an hour and a half before he gets here.

I am given a painkiller, but it brings no relief. I need all my strength to deal with this pain. I don't know how best to lie: All positions are equally uncomfortable. How much longer will it go on? Why doesn't anyone do anything?

Then suddenly Paul is there. He sits next to my bed and holds my hand; now I am no longer alone. A new attack makes everything around me fade away. I see a doctor, I hear "emergency," and the next moment I am being rolled into the operating room. Someone else, whose turn it actually was, is removed from the operating table: I have precedence. Condemned people are sometimes taken back to their cells just before their execution. Dying a thousand deaths. Thinking of the bullet. Has the bomb inside me already burst? Your Fallopian tubes can burst apart as a result of an ectopic pregnancy. You can bleed to death if that happens.

When I come round, I am lying in a room among all sorts of other people who have just had an operation. This must be the recovery room, although you imagine something a bit more comfortable when you hear that term. Here there is moaning, groaning, and crying. Two nurses are talking aloud about a patient they are finding tiresome. It seems as if my senses have been heightened. The sounds pound forcefully against me; everything is too much for me: the light, the noise, the sight of the other patients.

And what have they done with my abdomen? It is all blown up. I wish they would all keep quiet. I try to call one of the nurses; I want a painkiller, but my throat is painful and raw and my voice makes no sound. I have only ever had this experience in nightmares, where you try to call for help but no one can hear you. Why doesn't anyone come to check on me? Where is Paul?

Paul arrives when I've been back in the ward for a long time already. The nursing staff had told him to go home for a while, because I had to come round in the recovery room. I don't understand how they can send your loved one away when he should be there to hold your hand. And that the weakling simply allowed himself to be sent off. In the meantime I have received an injection for the pain. The doctor says that the operation was successful in saving my Fallopian tube and that they had used a laparoscope to remove the fetus from the tube. "We made an incision to allow the fetus to be born." As if he is giving me the good news of the birth of our child. Have I missed something? I surely haven't lain in a coma for months and now delivered a healthy baby? I ask the doctor to explain once again. Then I understand that they did not remove my Fallopian tube and that they had to make just a few small cuts in my abdomen. In a few days' time my abdomen, which was blown up with gas to enable the doctors to see better and give more space to work, will go down again. And in time the scars will hardly be visible.

One thing had surprised them: The pregnancy was not in the right Fallopian tube, as they had expected, but in the left one. I am not so surprised: After all, I had felt the pain on the left. Nonetheless it gives me a shock. My left Fallopian tube was my only good one. When I ask about the consequences, the doctor looks serious. After the good news comes the bad: "Your chances of a successful pregnancy have diminished considerably. The right Fallopian tube was already not completely clear. The scar tissue that will develop as a result of this operation will now reduce the clear passage in the left one as well. If you get pregnant again, you have an increased chance of another ectopic pregnancy."

Back home my eye falls on our luck-in-the-bedroom. The traitorous plant stands there glowing, as if nothing has happened. I want to cry bitterly, but can't, because any movement hurts my abdomen. I can only shed quiet tears, and that doesn't bring any relief. Joyce comes to visit and sits on a chair next to my bed. Because I cannot sit up yet, I look directly at her highly pregnant belly, which she would probably have preferred to leave behind on this occasion. It is like a comic scene from a tasteless B-grade movie. But I am not able to laugh yet either.

Our new house needs work. In a month's time we are getting married and holding a wedding dinner as a housewarming. I am trying to remember why we are doing all this, marrying and moving to that much-too-large, oppressively empty house. All I want to do is bury myself under the covers and sleep. The emptiness inside my belly seems to have taken over the whole of my body: I cannot feel anything at all, cannot think, don't want anything.

Only in the morning, when I wake up, when the day hasn't yet drawn a skin over my soul, do I feel naked and porous and even breathing is painful. I talk to myself: get up, go and wash, get dressed, get going. I am actually still supposed to be careful with lifting things and to take it easy, but once I have got myself out of my apathy, there is no stopping me. Removing curtains and carpets, stripping paint, removing nails, scrubbing, painting, recruiting friends and preparing food and drink for them, arranging a plumber, cleaning up, packing boxes, and booking a removal company. We do everything in the evening and over weekends, because during the day we have our normal jobs.

In the meantime the wedding has to be arranged. Consulting with Isabel and Natasha, our dedicated masters of ceremonies; organizing catering and the band; sending out invitations. A sharp abdominal pain reminds me regularly of the recent operation, but I do not want to know anything about it. I think my body is an unreliable instrument. It only destroys; I want to build things. A great deal emerges from my hands. I do everything mechanically and vacantly. Sometimes out of the blue I have an uncontrollable fit of crying. "I am so tired," I then complain to Paul, "I can't go on." But he, too, has his mind on the alterations. There is still so much to be done before the wedding. And so we go on from where we left off.

Natasha and her boyfriend have also just bought a house in the same town. As we are busy painting, they come by, after signing the title deed for their house. Natasha takes me to one side. She has to tell me something, she whispers conspiratorially. She confides in me, extremely nervously, that she is madly in love with someone else. She is like a snorting horse, on the point of breaking loose and galloping away. She does not want to live here at all, and she does not want to marry this man. The thought of having to start a family with him in that house makes her feel as if she is suffocating. She does not want to bury herself alive, she wants to leave, give up her job, break off her relationship, and run away with her new flame.

"But then why have you just bought the house?" I ask.

"I'm wondering about that, too. As soon as I'd signed my name, I knew for certain I shouldn't have done it. It felt completely wrong. I have to tell him, I have to reverse it, it cannot go through."

A few days later she comes to tell me that she has worked it all out. They are going to resell the house, she has resigned from her job, and she will soon be going abroad. She looks like a different person. She is a bundle of passion and energy. I look at her with a mixture of admiration and jealousy. To think that you can free yourself from your shackles like that in just a few days! I wish that I could leave everything behind. But what I would like most to leave behind me is the gnawing pain in my abdomen, my tiredness, and my inability to enjoy things. I would also like to glow like that, to be in love, to break free, to live. But I am not in a hurry for another boyfriend, another job, another house, or another country. I cannot free myself of my shackles, because it is my own body that has for the second time given me such a raw deal. My enemy is inside me and is undermining the happiness in my life from within.

"And how are you doing?" Natasha asks, suddenly concerned when she sees my blank expression.

"I am going to get married and bury myself alive in this provincial town."

One of our witnesses takes his role very seriously. He is happy to be a witness at our wedding, but then he wants to be sure that we have a good relationship. He knows about our problems with the pregnancies. He is aware of my complaints about Paul after the miscarriage. He thinks that I look dreadfully unhappy and has the impression that once again Paul is not supporting or looking after me as he should. We should go to counseling together, in his view. We cannot simply get over this type of drama by working ourselves into a frenzy and acting as if nothing is wrong.

Yet that is precisely what I want now. I do not want to deal at length with the fact that a normal pregnancy is even less likely. I find the idea so unacceptable that I don't feel able to cope with it yet. First let me finally get over the pain in my abdomen, let us get the house fixed up, let us get the wedding behind us. I have no desire to talk about our relationship. I am relieved simply to be able to remain standing. And that our friends are there for us with practical, concrete help with the house alterations and organizing the wedding. And that Paul is so handy that he is able to lay a beautiful wooden floor and plaster walls himself. The witness looks unconvinced.

Everything is fine with our relationship, I tell him reassuringly but without much conviction. We have been together ten years now, mostly happy and sometimes unhappy, like now. Is that a reason not to get married? The witness looks even more doubtful. I don't think it sounds particularly romantic either.

Yet we have both learned something since the last setback. Paul now knows that he can avoid a great deal of moaning on my part by not hanging around the bar during times of crisis. I now know that in emergency situations Paul does not sense what I need. And so I need to be very clear about this myself. When I was discharged from the hospital after the operation, I instructed him to stay home for the first few days to look after me. I explained to him that he needed to come and check on me at regular intervals, say nice things to me, and hold my hand. When he did not come often enough, I had a bell placed next to my bed that I could use to call him. After that we were both happy: I because I was getting what I needed, and he because I was not angry and did not moan.

I would naturally prefer it if Paul thought of these things himself. When you are feeling weak, it is difficult to have to keep on running the show yourself, but Paul has other characteristics that balance up against this. His sense of humor and his ability to put things into perspective remain untouched, even in difficult times. I can then use them to help myself. One needs not only support, but also distraction. Paul does not give me a chance to sit down in despair. And painting your house can also have a very therapeutic effect.

The witness is not very convinced, but he gives us the benefit of the doubt.

On our wedding day I look radiant. I wear a bright red off-the-shoulder dress with a fitted bodice and a wide gathered skirt that is short in the front and longer at the back. I had to have the dress taken in twice. First because it was intended to be used with a pregnant belly, and then once more because the stress of the past few months had resulted in my weight continuing to fall to well under my normal level. But this morning I woke up without any pain, without feeling exhausted, without tears. I feel like a child having a birthday, eagerly anticipating what the day might bring.

Isabel and Natasha buzz around me like motherly bees. They help me into my sexy lingerie and use a wet finger to clean some stray makeup from my face at the last minute. My mother is nervously fiddling with the flowers woven into the hair of our nieces and bridesmaids, who look unbelievably cute in their white dresses.

In good times and in bad, we solemnly promise each other today. All at once this worn-out expression touches me deeply. Paul does not restrict himself to the usual "I do" but says emphatically: "I most definitely do." I glance at him to see whether he is making fun of the situation, but he is serious. My eyes fill. I had never imagined that we would both take this ceremony so seriously. My hand trembles when Paul slips the ring onto my finger: a pretty ring in three shades of gold with a small diamond in the middle.

As we walk out of the town hall, a shower of rice is thrown over us. I keep the grains that fall onto my hair and clothes in place as long as possible so that their magic power can pervade my being.

My mother has organized a reception at her home. My great-uncle, a retired pastry chef, has made us an impressive wedding cake. My father gives a loving speech before the champagne corks pop. Even though my parents have been divorced for years and never officially remarried, they stand next to one another, both moved.

The caterers arrive far too late to the dinner, so everyone is already fairly tipsy by the time we start eating. During the festivities Paul's family perform a lovely wild song. His brother strums crazily on the guitar. Dick strides across the stage screaming and waving his arms wildly. His dragging foot is the only visible evidence of his stroke, but here it looks like a conscious act. A broadly grinning Irene and her even more Mongol-looking fiancé accompany the musical violence with a civilized but a-rhythmic jingling on the tambourine. Gwen, a former teacher, tries in vain to declaim the text in an understandable way. Isabel is looking after the guests, who are still arriving, and the gifts. She walks up and down nervously as if it is her own wedding.

70

Later in the evening a great rock 'n' roll band plays. To my delight I see that Natasha is flirting shamelessly with the singer in the band. This is exactly what I had hoped for: not an evening of pleasant anecdotes, but a real party with music, flirting, and dancing. I dance the whole evening, too, without getting tired. Paul watches me lovingly. The dolphin on my bare shoulder dances joyously with us. Reach for the stars!

CHAPTER FOUR

ISABEL IS PREGNANT,

or

How I Become Estranged from My Best Friend

Isabel is pregnant. Suddenly I understand why she had announced so earnestly that she wanted to tell me something. With anyone else I would have smelled a rat immediately, but not with Isabel. It is not all that long since things ended abruptly with her last boyfriend. She was dreadfully upset about it.

I don't know how I should react. I stammer some words of congratulations—or was it an accident? No, it was wanted. She had been on vacation with her new boyfriend during the summer, and they decided then that they wanted a child. And it happened just like that. She is somewhat overwhelmed, she says; she hadn't expected it to happen so quickly.

I am completely taken aback. I've known Isabel longer than I've known Paul. Our friendship began as a sort of love affair. If I had been a lesbian, or if she had been a man, she could have been the love of my life. We have the same background, the same interests, the same sense of humor. I know all about her boyfriends and her problems in love. I know her whole family, and she mine. We talk about everything. Or so I thought.

I was not even aware that she wanted a child at this stage. She had never mentioned it. Not that she didn't want children at all, but they could come later. She is also a few years younger than me. I had problems getting pregnant, she had problems with her relationships. She always fell for men who made her unhappy. She found nice men dull; they bored her too quickly. Noam seemed to me to be a nice man. I had no idea that she took her relationship with him so seriously.

It's as if the love of my life has just run out on me. I feel betrayed and excluded. Sidelined. Angry. Jealous. Of Noam, with whom she has become intimate so unexpectedly, and of the pregnancy that she has had dropped into her lap. It is now five years since Paul and I decided we would like children. Five years is a long time. And Isabel gets pregnant just like that.

Painful telephone conversations follow in which we try to talk things through. I am not the only one who feels left in the lurch. She feels hurt by my excessive reaction to the news of her pregnancy. Why is it so surprising that she is pregnant? Isn't she allowed to be? She had wanted to tell me, even though it wasn't easy. But when and how should she have done so? I was constantly preoccupied with myself. I could surely have asked her myself. I could surely have seen it coming, if my eyes had been open. She is already thirty-one, after all, and has just finished her studies. So it's surely not such an unusual step.

I reproach her for not having told me anything. If she only tells me when her heart is broken, how am I supposed to tell that she has already taken three huge steps with the next man in the meantime? She should have prepared me for this. Particularly since she knows how sensitive I am about the topic. Or did she simply want to spare me? That would be completely unforgivable. You do not spare a true friend.

To celebrate Isabel's finishing graduate school, a group of us meet for dinner. Isabel avoids me. I am closer to crying than to laughing. I go and sit next to Noam. I have to brace myself to congratulate him on Isabel's pregnancy. "You didn't expect that, did you?" he replies, laughing. The note of triumph I hear in his voice undoes all my resolve. I stumble outside and burst into tears. Noam comes after me and asks what is wrong. I get myself under control again and say to him that the news of the pregnancy had really surprised me. That I had had no idea that they wanted a child together.

"Isabel and I considered this to be something between the two of us. It is something intimate, which you don't want to share with just anyone," Noam replies. His reaction pours oil on fire. I am now seething inside. Who does he think he is with his "Isabel and I"? He's bloody well new on the scene! Isabel is the friend I have shared joys and sorrows with for fifteen years!

How dare he reduce me to "just anyone"! I would like to give him a beating, but instead I shut up. In silence we go back in.

I also insulted Noam, I gather from another of the numerous difficult telephone conversations with Isabel. After all, we had met regularly, we had eaten and laughed together. They both thought that I liked him. And now it seems that I had regarded him as an unimportant halfway station, a temporary boyfriend to provide some comfort.

They themselves had created that impression, I retort. She had never talked about him as the new love of her life. She wasn't living with him. How was I supposed to know it was so serious?

Her accusation that I was so self-absorbed, that I had paid no attention to her hits home. Because she is right. Since my ectopic pregnancy I have hardly had time for her. First there was the operation, then the move, then the house, and finally the wedding. Isabel came to visit while I was still in bed, helped with the painting, and was master of ceremonies. There has been far too much one-way traffic.

Her other accusation also hits the nail on the head. To my mind she shouldn't be having a child yet. I should have been first. At the same time would also have been fine. But this I can't accept. I find the sight of a pregnant woman I don't even know difficult enough. When they are friends of mine, it's even worse. But when it is my best friend who is pregnant, it is simply intolerable. Her pregnancy mirrors my loss. Even if she had prepared me for it, I would have had to dig deep within myself to go through this with her. Since she didn't do so, let her share this intimate experience with Noam. After all it is something between the two of them.

I once had a romantic notion of the ideal love relationship: that you are able to share everything with one another, that you understand one another without words, that you melt together body and soul. But then I was still a child. I have long since accepted that you cannot share everything with one single person, and certainly not with a man. Many men do not have the sensitivity to place themselves in another's position. The attraction in my relationship with Paul lies precisely in the fact that we are so different from one another. The distance maintains the tension, and that keeps the sex good. For intimacy I had Isabel. This is now in the past. We phone one another occasionally, but uncomfortable silences develop in our conversations. We do not know exactly what to talk about. The sense of confidentiality has disappeared.

Am I naïve! The expectation that best friends are able to share everything with one another was another childish idea. In fact, Noam is right: Having a child is something between the two of them. It is their child; I am indeed on the periphery. There are always adjustments when friends have children.

Such a dramatic change automatically results in friendships becoming slightly less important.

Relationships run down, as does life as a whole. In the end you die, and that you do alone. The closest friendships develop when you are in your teens or twenties. That is when you are at your most open, when the need to share is greatest. When people start long-term relationships, they spend more time with their partner and the friendships move to second place. When they eventually have children, they have even less time available for their friends. Now and again they still see friends who also have children, and the children can play together while the parents chat about their kids. Personal conversations become rare. You no longer bother your friend with your problems. You take them to a psychiatrist, or keep them to yourself.

Soon I'll be all alone with Paul, unhappy, bitter and lonely, without children, without friends, without Isabel. And eventually, possibly, without Paul. One day he will have had enough of my somber moods.

CHAPTER FIVE

THE IVF CIRCUS,

or

How I Am Moved by Quivering Raspberries

The waiting room is full of pregnant women. Birth announcement cards are hanging everywhere. Perhaps this pointed display of fertility is intended to put us in an optimistic frame of mind. With IVF—in vitro fertilization—all these desirable things are in the offing for you, too! But I am intimidated by them, and they make me feel anxious. I want to get out.

I am just back from a visit to the book fair in Zimbabwe. It was not only an interesting trip workwise. My ego, too, grew at least ten centimeters. It was an erotically charged week. My heartache and the pain in my belly had disappeared; my body belonged to me again. I even felt attractive, and this apparently radiated from me. I had completely forgotten what that felt like. I was tempted to be unfaithful. Paul would never need to know. Who knew what he did while I was away? You only live once; before you know it, you are old and ugly and berating yourself for having lived like a chaste nun. After Paul's affair with Maria, I'd declared now and again that I still had the right of revenge, but now this has exceeded its statutory limits.

Sometimes a potential lover asks me invitingly: "Why do you actually want a child? If you have love to spare, why don't you take a lover?" And he gives me a seductive "come hither" look. I enjoy that kind of attention. I like flirting and being provocative. I enjoy playing the game of enticement. But when push comes to shove, I still prefer to crawl into bed with Paul. His body is my favorite destination. I know every inch of it. There are other attractive places, but this is the one I always want to come back to. Even now that my fertile periods are ruling our sex life, we have not allowed this to reduce our pleasure in bed in any way. This is a gift from heaven, as I know it could just as easily cause the joy of sex to be lost, because you associate it only with doomed attempts at reproduction.

The relationship between sex and reproduction had never really made much of an impression on me. I was bored stiff when my parents gave us sex education. The run-up to their sudden openness about the birds and the bees and the sperm and the eggs was rather more interesting. My brother and sister and I and two neighborhood friends formed a secret sex club. None of us were sexually mature yet. Our simple games were innocent, but still exciting in a childlike way.

We drew our inspiration from pictures from an adult magazine that my brother was able to get his hands on. Together we developed a game, with a full set of rules. We took turns throwing the dice and, depending on the picture on which you landed, you had to do something with someone, like kiss them in various places or sit on top of one another in positions similar to those in the photos. I was just settling into a complicated position with one of the other club members when my father came in unexpectedly and caught us in the act. He did not get angry—my parents were open-minded—but he ended the game at once. We had to put our clothes back on and accompany him to the living room immediately. There he began, in my mother's presence—and on this occasion she said not a word against him—to give us a sleep-inducing explanation of what mothers and fathers do together to make a baby. It was clear that this functional description was intended for grown-ups, and I couldn't understand why he was bothering us children with it.

Later I was given sex education once again at school. That was a bit more interesting, because our teacher had devised a system to allow pupils to ask questions anonymously. We could put folded notes into a plastic container on his desk. He promised to answer all questions, and we didn't need a second invitation. We questioned him from top to bottom, and without flinching or blushing he told us how often he did it with his wife, that his wife indeed also had red hair down there, and approximately how long his thingy was, unaroused and in erection. Very quickly there were complaints from parents, and the container disappeared from his desk. But by then we already knew pretty much all we wanted to know.

80

Around the same time—we were about twelve years old— we also held school parties in garages, from which the parents discreetly absented themselves. We filled the evenings largely by playing musical chairs without any chairs. The boys formed an inner circle, and the girls walked around them in time to the music. When the music stopped, you had to French kiss the boy you had stopped in front of. Then the music started up, and off you went again. Of course plenty of cheating went on, so the parties were nowhere near as much fun for everyone. But I was always very lucky. And not only in love, mind you.

My father said I was a Sunday's child, and all things considered I still am today. I am good-looking; I am healthy; I have a partner, lots of friends, good relations with my family, a good education, a nice job, and no money worries. No children, it's true, but that also has its advantages. There are many people without children who are perfectly happy with their lives. Possibly far happier than many people who do have children, with all the worries, responsibility, and lack of freedom that they bring. And would I be able to take such nice long trips if I had children? Would I still be able to go out and dance, drink and talk deep into the night? And isn't it slowly becoming time for the next step in my career, now that I've been doing the same work at the same publisher for three years?

In college a female professor mentioned during a lecture, in the presence of a whole group of students, that she had been unable to have children. Otherwise she would have become a housewife, she said, because that had been her sole ambition. When she didn't have any luck with children, she devoted herself to science. As luck would have it, she was very successful in that department.

I was impressed by her story, even though at that stage I still had no idea what it meant not to be able to have children. Until then I had associated infertility with pitiful, dried-up women, but the professor was pretty and lively, dressed elegantly and sexily, and furthermore enjoyed international recognition in her field. She had everything that I admired in a woman, and now she appeared to be human and wise as well. She told her story very calmly and in a neutral tone, as if to illustrate that life does not always go the way we want it to, but that this does not always mean disaster. On the contrary, failure can be a building block for success. I would also be able to be successful, if I didn't keep sinking deeper into the quagmire of my frustrated desire for a child. I wonder, am I not being incredibly stupid now, starting off on the slippery path of IVF as well? Am I not throwing away my best years?

Paul has no such doubts. Nor is he as ambitious as I am. He wants to enjoy his work, earn enough money, and have time to play his guitar, play tennis, and go out with friends. But he finds the idea of a future without children rather bare. "Then everything stays the same," he says. "I also want to experience life from another perspective."

I notice how sure he is of himself. Two scenarios rise up before me if I let my imagination go. One: Paul leaving me to have children with someone else. Two: Paul staying with me, but silently blaming me for not being able to give him children, so our relationship becomes soured.

I find both options insupportable, but not unimaginable. If you really want children, that desire can become stronger than your love for your partner. And there is nothing wrong with him; he is quite able to have children. The problem lies with me. According to the doctor, the reason for my Fallopian tube being blocked is an earlier infection, which could have been caused by one of my succession of partners. Paul knows this, but he has never complained about it. If he did, I would be annoyed with him. Those adventures were before his time. I do not regret them; there was no way I could have foreseen these consequences. Still, I know that in moments of weakness he could point an accusing finger at me, and he doesn't. If he wants it so badly, I will do my level best to give him children. Anyway, I don't trust my sudden relish for a future without children. Perhaps I am trying to arm myself against new disappointments.

"IVF is generally used in cases like yours, where blocked Fallopian tubes are what prevent a normal pregnancy from occurring. With IVF you can leave the Fallopian tubes out of the equation, since the egg is placed directly in the womb after fertilization."

It all sounds very simple and completely logical. I have no problem with the fact that the fertilization is done artificially; it is still our own ingredients that are put together. It is irrelevant whether this happens in my tubes or outside of them; the result is what is important: a normal pregnancy and a child. After all the examinations, I am used to spreading my legs for a doctor, and Paul has also had some experience with coming in a container.

"The treatment is generally felt to be burdensome," warns the lady doing our initial interview. We ask about the success rate. "The chance of a pregnancy is about twenty percent per attempt. That may not seem like much, but it is comparable with the natural chances of a pregnancy in women without complications. Many women get pregnant within three attempts. That number is also paid for by most medical insurance plans."

She explains to us the technicalities of what we would each have to do. Normally one egg ripens each month in a woman's cycle, but you have thousands in reserve. With in vitro fertilization, injections with natural hormones are used to produce a number of ripe eggs at the same time in order to increase the chances of successful fertilization. Ultrasounds and blood tests are used to carefully track the process of ripening. When the eggs are ripe, a needle is used to suck them up. In the meantime the man has to produce semen on the spot, and the two are brought together. Then there is a few days' waiting to see whether the eggs are fertilized and whether cell division starts occurring. If this happens, one or more of the fertilized eggs are put back into the uterus. And then there is two weeks' waiting to see whether the embryo becomes properly implanted.

When we leave, we are given a huge pile of folders and information and prescriptions. I am overwhelmed. When I hand the prescriptions in at the pharmacy the next day, I can scarcely carry the two large paper bags I receive. They are bursting with large and small injections; different size containers of liquid, in various colors with labels that say Decapeptyl, Humegon, Pregnyl; needles, large and small, thick and thin, some attached to syringes and others not; bandages; gauze; and alcohol.

Usually I only go to the drug store for a box of aspirin or a pregnancy test. I lay out this awe-inspiring loot for Paul, hooting with laughter: Look, this is the equipment for producing our future child. We study the contents and divide up the tasks.

The small injections with Decapeptyl go into my stomach; I will give them to myself. I've never had to inject myself before, but I tell myself people with diabetes do it their whole lives long. I find it a bit nerve-racking the first few times, but I soon get used to it and it hardly hurts at all. This preparatory phase normally takes two weeks, but in our case, together with the examination, it lasts six. The annual visit to the Frankfurt book fair also falls during this period, and this is a very intensive and important week. I take a small supply of injections with me, and for the sake of our objective I try not to drink any alcohol in the evenings, which is a real sacrifice in this environment. Going out to eat together, but also to drink, is the major form of relaxation after a hard day's work. On various occasions I am asked if I am perhaps pregnant, when once again I order a mineral water, to which I react a little awkwardly. The hormones make me feel unstable. I have difficulty maintaining a businesslike and efficient appearance.

There is one appointment in particular that makes me really uncomfortable. A fanatical literary agent is trying to sell me a book entitled *The Myth of Motherhood.* I keep her at bay: "Something like that doesn't fit into our line," which is, in fact, quite true. But she is not going to be stopped. "Women are forced into motherhood. Women are told that without children they will never know fulfillment. There is no such thing as the instinct of motherhood; that is something that was invented by men. Women who are unable to bear children feel that they are failures and go to the most extreme lengths to try to comply with the myth. They allow themselves to be operated on, they inject themselves full of hormones, they allow themselves to be pushed around. Do you have any idea how many women these days subject themselves to IVF treatment? IVF is one of the most objectionable developments of our time. It is an invention that supports and maintains the myth of motherhood." I think of the tubes full of hormones in my hotel fridge. This evening I will be giving myself a shot once again.

"Is the author not seriously underestimating women if she thinks that they are so stupid as to let themselves be talked into the desire to have a child?" I try to argue. I am aware that this has nothing to do with the author's views. The discussion is not about the book; it is about us. This woman quite clearly is personally involved in the subject, as am I. Where else does her acerbity come from?

"No, it is not that women are stupid. They are just so unbelievably sensitive to what men want from them and to what is expected of them, instead of making conscious choices for themselves."

I leave for my next appointment in a cloud of confusion. Am I doing it for Paul? In part, yes. If he didn't want it so much, I certainly wouldn't have gone so far. But it would be really tragic if I was doing it only for him. Naturally I also want a child by him—although I find myself wondering more and more often how much exactly. Motherhood does not particularly attract me. My heart does not melt at the sight of a baby. I find mothers with bags under their eyes trudging along behind strollers an unattractive sight.

But I know only too well what it is like to be full of expectation. I know how painful the feeling of loss is when you have a miscarriage. Pregnant bellies make my heart sink. Evidently I am not yet able to accept that I will not have any children. So I assume that I do have a desire to have a child. What point is there in thinking about it anymore? If I did, I would remain eternally thrashing around in my own doubts. Perhaps my greatest problem is, in fact, that I have too much time to doubt. I believe in impulsive decisions; I think that all important decisions are taken with the heart. But my heart has too much time. This fills it with doubt.

Other people don't have to consider endlessly whether or not they want a child. They also don't know what they are getting into and whether it will be worth the effort. At a certain moment they simply take a shot and see what happens. I am also taking a shot, except that in my case it is costing me a lot of time and effort, but in the end it's all the same. You do what you have to do. And now I have to do a round of IVF. Motherhood will be something to worry about later, and the myth of motherhood doesn't concern me in the least.

When I get back home, it's time for the big injections with the thick needles. Turn and turn about, first in the left buttock and then in the right. This is Paul's responsibility; he learned how to do it at the hospital.

"May I come inside you?" he asks half-lewdly before he plunges the needle into my buttock.

"Yes, do, deeper, deeper!" I shout back as I stick my backside up.

I am still not able to take jokes from others on this subject. I am sorry I wasn't able to keep it completely to myself. One of my friends calls IVF "ordering a baby from the hospital." A good friend, whose coarse humor I generally enjoy immensely, says to me: "So, soon you'll be getting a Mengele baby?"

Without any anesthetic, they put a thick needle right through the wall of my vagina to remove the ripened eggs from my abdomen. The withdrawal seems to take forever. In the meantime Paul is allowed to have fun masturbating in a special room with a bed and titillating reading material. Men say it's no picnic to have to come on command, but at least it doesn't hurt. My insides are punched full of holes; it feels like a form of torture. It appears that some women feel absolutely nothing. I am evidently extremely sensitive.

The harvest is good: twelve eggs. Now we have to wait to see whether or not the fertilization is successful. If I was religious, I could pray for it to go well. I once read about an old woman in China who was so afraid of airplanes that she mentally accompanied her daughter's or granddaughter's flight to America. She flew with them in her mind and supported the wings to prevent the plane from crashing. In a similar manner I send my thoughts out to the hospital, and I concentrate on the joining of Paul's sperm and my eggs somewhere in a little container or tube in the laboratory. Come on, guys, make a real orgy of it!

A few days later the liberating telephone call comes: Four eggs have been fertilized, among which are two embryos of outstanding quality, according to the people at the laboratory. I thought an egg was an egg and sperm were sperm, but it now appears that the combination of ours has produced embryos of outstanding quality. I almost feel proud, just like the time I received a compliment about my uterus.

Before they are put into my womb, we want to have a look at the two embryos. They are projected onto a television screen. They look like raspberries, two little round things made up of tiny beads, which are the divided cells. I am moved by their awkward trembling, as if they already have something human about them. When they are put back inside me, I feel almost nothing. I do experience it as a solemn moment, though. Once it's been done, we are left alone. I must remain on my back for a quarter of an hour, and Paul holds my hand tightly. We are a little dumbstruck. What can you say, what should you think? Absolutely nothing is certain yet, but still, there is the start of new life in my womb once again. And with it hope is born once more.

The next day I develop a high temperature and severe abdominal pains. Even the smallest movement is agony, and I am terrified when it appears that we have to take the car and drive all the way to the hospital an hour away. We selected that hospital because it was close enough to my office; I could arrange my many visits around my working hours. Up to now I had been very happy with our choice. I have never been treated as well in any hospital as I have by the IVF team there. Now I curse the distance. Every time Paul accelerates, brakes, or takes a corner, I moan in misery.

In the hospital everything takes forever. Blood tests, ultrasound, cultivation, internal examination. It's probably an infection of the ovary, says the gynecologist. This has a negative effect on fertility, but this is the last thing on my mind at the moment. I feel much too awful for that. I am given a prescription for an antibiotic and for Flagyl to fight the infection. Afterward I lie on my back in bed with a high temperature for three days, my hands on my abdomen, waiting for the time and the pain to pass.

Isabel comes to visit. We have not seen one another since our estrangement. Her visit is intended to show that she is still my friend. This does me good, even though I have no idea how we are to give form to our friendship now. Her pregnant belly is beginning to show. I try to say something light and amusing about it, as a forced token of recognition. Fortunately she does not take it any further. She has some women's magazines with her. We both find them the height of self-indulgence and relaxation. She makes me tea. We don't talk much. What should we talk about? Our experiences are diametrically opposed to one another, and we are both extremely absorbed in them. She has the internally focused absence of mind of a pregnant woman who is full of the wonder that is developing in her belly. Whereas in my belly I feel only pain.

Will the two embryos survive this dreadful experience? It's almost impossible to imagine that they could. The doctors say that such a severe infection practically never occurs as a result of IVF treatment. Just my luck! Next time, they promise, they will give me a preventive antibiotic "screen," as they put it in graphic terms. Does that mean they already regard this attempt as doomed to failure? I feel none of the familiar signs of pregnancy; my breasts are not full. But perhaps it's still too early for this. I haven't started another period yet, and that should have happened by now. Someone tells me that a high temperature has no effect on embryos; they are implanted the way they are precisely to protect them against that sort of influence from outside. So maybe . . .

A month and a half of feeling unstable because of the hormones: for nothing. Almost daily doses of blood being taken and ultrasounds being done: a waste of time. The anxiety about the injection: pointless. Lying in bed for days as if paralyzed: for nothing. Two long weeks of waiting and hoping, even though you know better: simply the usual start of another period with the same old severe cramps. They couldn't even freeze the remaining two eggs; they turned out not to be top quality after all.

I hear nothing further from Isabel either. There appears to be an unexpected reason for this: She was admitted to the hospital with an acute kidney infection. In the meantime, she has been given a course of antibiotics and is home again. I consult the medical encyclopedia. Such infections often occur in pregnant women and, provided they are treated promptly, there is no threat to the baby. The danger is thus minimal, but Isabel got a huge fright. So now it is my turn to prove my friendship.

I go to visit her, take along some light reading matter and make tea. She tells me how scared she was of losing her child. As if it is a unique experience. As if her anxiety is worse than my reality. My twins would have been three years old; the child from my second pregnancy would have been born already if it had not implanted itself in the wrong place. My latest dream child has just been nipped in the bud. I look at her belly, which has become considerably larger since the last time. In due course she will simply have her baby. I pour her another cup of tea.

I get really annoyed with people who see everything in terms of their Personal Disaster. People who have something wrong with them and seize every opportunity to sigh, "At least you are healthy." Lonely folk who end every conversation with, "At least you have a partner." In the face of their suffering, everyone else's is reduced to nothing. And now I am busy turning into one of those frustrated people. Don't moan; at least you have (or will soon have, as the case may be) a child. I haven't said it out loud yet, but I'm getting close.

I ward off complaints by others with stories about how it could have been much worse. If someone complains about a difficult delivery, I tell them in vivid detail about my sister-in-law's experience in a backward hospital in Poland. My eldest brother was a diplomat there. When his wife's waters broke, they drove by car through a rainy Warsaw to the elite hospital for foreigners and the Polish upper class. They got lost. After a nerve-racking drive through the city, labor was so far advanced that they stopped at the first hospital they came across. There she received no preferential treatment. It was a rough introduction to the life of the ordinary Poles. My brother was not allowed to be present at the delivery, for reasons of hygiene. He had to watch from behind a screen as his wife appeared to be slaughtered like a pig. There was not a single medical indication that a Caesarean birth was necessary; she had brought her previous three children into the world without any problem. Afterward the child was wrapped up tightly and taken away to another part of the hospital. When my sister-in-law protested, she was given an injection to knock her out. My brother was sent away. My sister-in-law came round and, extremely upset, asked for her husband and her child. Once again she was given an injection to calm her down. It is a wonderful story to tell. Always puts them in their place. But I am aware that my pleasure is derived from the aggressive desire to reprimand the complainers.

Nobody gains anything from comparing their suffering with someone else's. Even my situation might be enviable to another person. A friend of mine is jealous of me because I have been pregnant a couple of times. She has also been trying for years, but absolutely nothing has happened in her case. They don't know the reason and are unable to do anything. "You at least know that you can get pregnant," she says. "That in itself is a lot more than I have."

For some women it's absolutely no fun being pregnant. The delivery can be a traumatic experience. Women can be confused and depressed after the birth of their child. The child can also have all sorts of things wrong with it. Everyone has setbacks, and everyone has different levels of what she is able to bear. Some people survive humiliations that no one should have to go through, without losing their spirit. Compared with the torture they have endured, my setbacks pale into insignificance.

I know this only too well. But heart and mind are unfortunately not always in sync. At times one's emotions charge ahead, and at others they trudge along behind one's mind. Sometimes they lose the path and run ridiculous circles round one another, until you can no longer work out who is trying to keep up with whom. That's the position I am in now, an inextricable ball of misery. Like laundry in a dryer, I keep turning in the same tight circle around my empty middle. Dented, crumpled, small. How can I get out of here? I want to stretch out and feel the wind on me, smell the outside air, see the horizon.

An older colleague with whom I get on well confides his story to me. Twice he and his wife had children who were not fully developed when they were born—first a little boy whom they named Christian, then a little girl named Suzanne. "With today's techniques they could have saved them," he says. At the time he really didn't know how to deal with the dramatic circumstances.

Shortly after that he was also told by the doctor that his wife had multiple sclerosis. The doctor did not tell her about it.

My colleague did not dare tell her either, after the heavy blows she had already had to endure. Of course she realized in time, and things got completely out of hand. They were separated for a while, but in the end they sorted everything out, because they loved one another deeply. They still find it sad that they have no children, but they have come to accept it. If someone at work celebrates the birth of a child, he is glad for them. He knows that having a baby is something very special and does not begrudge anyone such a gift.

To me, his attitude is one of superhuman generosity. Someone suffering because he is unemployed can surely not be truly happy for someone else who has just landed his dream job. Someone who has just lost her mother is not going to give a willing ear to your complaints about your own mother's rudeness. Someone who is getting over a broken relationship cannot bear the sight of love-struck couples. Someone else's luck can burn like sharp sun on unprotected skin. If you are exposed to it for too long, your skin is ruined before you know it.

"How do you get over something like that?" I ask my colleague, in the hope of receiving a wise lesson of life.

"It was years ago. You learn to live with it. But don't think that you ever get over it completely. The scars remain; they become part of you. Sometimes they itch, and sometimes they even tear open again, for example when you are asked the inevitable question whether you have children. I often say no, just to be done with it. My wife has a problem with this. She thinks that by doing it I deny the existence of Christian and Suzanne. And of course, she is right."

A set of twins is born in Paul's family. Gwen, who had been so thrilled at the time of my first pregnancy, has become a grand-mother at last. She is at least as proud of the twins as Simon and Lois are. A few years after he had his sterilization reversed, their hospital saga was crowned with success.

Naturally we are thrilled for them. Obviously we go to admire the babies. They are two unbelievably tiny little things, lying side by side in one crib. We compliment the beaming parents. We ask politely about sleeping and eating patterns, because we know that's what new parents like to talk about. We give presents and have a celebratory tea. We look at the nursery and say that it is lovely. When we leave, I see a twin stroller standing in the hallway. There was a time when I never even knew they existed, but you get them in all kinds and sizes. Wide ones, so that the children can sit next to one another, and long ones, in which they sit one behind the other. There is also a long version, where the children sit facing one another. I discovered these varieties of twin carriages just after my mis-carriage. The city suddenly appeared to be full of them.

After the visit to the new babies, we call in on Gwen and Dick, who live nearby. When Gwen asks me excitedly as we come in what I think of her grandchildren, I burst into tears. Her face clouds over. I wish I could control myself better. I am a spell breaker.

You must not keep wallowing in your grief, you must work through it and accept it, they say. The words are spouted so easily, especially when they apply to someone else. You should talk it out, but with whom? Your partner is a man and cannot identify with a woman. Your friends are pregnant themselves and living in another world. Those who have suffered the same fate understand, but you can't rely on them. Just as you are about to go and moan about the swelling wombs around you, they themselves suddenly announce their joyous news.

Perhaps I should go to a psychiatrist after all. Spend more time with the white-jacket brigade. If they could make me get pregnant with words, I would go immediately, but what will I get out of all the jabbering? A psychiatrist can of course help you to gain more insight into yourself. But I have no lack of self-insight. Talking does not solve anything in my case; at the most it brings some relief. But you can gain relief in other ways, too. A good fit of crying can bring relief; writing in your diary can make you feel better. I have been going through large numbers of tissues and notebooks since I stopped baring my heart to others. Playing sports also helps heal. A friend of mine, who was in therapy for years after almost dying of anorexia nervosa, swears by marathon running. "A round of running costs nothing and helps more than all the psychia-trists put together."

I do not like running and so have to find something else to improve my fitness. I want to get into shape for my second IVF attempt. It appears like an unassailable mountain, but I can't just leave it at that. After a car accident, the best thing to do is to get back behind the wheel at once.

CHAPTER SIX

WITH THE COURAGE OF DESPAIR,

or

My Longing for the End

"People think they have a right to a child. If they are unable to have children, they appeal to the medical profession, expecting instant satisfaction." I don't know anyone who gets these results, and certainly do not count myself among that rare species. But my brother-in-law obviously does—why else would he say this to me? Friends and acquaintances ask one another—with annoying self-confidence—when they should "have" their child. They fine-tune the moment carefully to fit in with their career planning. They look for a crib before the child has even been conceived. They know that not everyone is able to have a child at the drop of a hat, but are sure *they* will have no problem. And, as unfair as it seems, this is usually the case. You wish it was a bit more difficult.

Sometimes I feel just like someone who went through a winter of famine during a war. The spoiled postwar generation has absolutely no idea what hunger is! But what good does my worldly wisdom do me, except make me even more bitter? At most it brings me to the painful realization that there's nothing I can do.

That is why my brother-in-law's remark infuriates me so. I know perfectly well that you can't have everything the way you want it. I know that better than he does. It's easy for him to talk. His wife—my younger sister—has just told me that she is pregnant with her second child. She sees my malicious look and in a protective reflex action pulls her jersey over her bulging belly. I feel like the evil witch standing at the cradle of their future child. I must get away.

On the way home, I think about how I could have countered his remark. As a budding doctor, he may have been able to identify with this comparison: People with heart problems are eager to make use of a bypass in order to be able to live longer. IVF is also a form of assistance to get around a malfunctioning Fallopian tube. It makes it possible to fulfill the desire to reproduce, a desire that to my mind is just as legitimate as the desire to use modern techniques to lengthen your life. In both situations quality of life is improved.

But why should I enter into a discussion about this? If his intention is to have a theoretical chat about who does and who does not have the right to medical assistance in order to get pregnant, then he doesn't have to do it with me but with his colleagues at the hospital. No doubt they find it interesting to deliberate about the cost-benefit ratio, the rules and the ethical boundaries that should be set. I do not. I simply want a child.

When I phone my sister to congratulate her on the birth of their second child, she asks how our second IVF attempt went. Unsuccessful once again, better next time, I summarize briefly.

She feels really sorry for us. Her sympathy, just after giving birth herself, mind you, moves me, and I decide after all to go and visit her and the baby soon. Two years ago I was present, without any reservations, at the birth of her first child. My role was much smaller than for Anna's delivery, but once again I found the occasion as magical as it was impressive. I hoped to be able to take part more often and offered myself as a volunteer to my friends, but after my second unsuccessful pregnancy, no one took me up on the offer again. I didn't repeat it, either.

When I tell my older brother that we were unsuccessful, he says by way of comfort: "I know a couple who also tried for a very long time, and when they stopped the treatment she suddenly got pregnant. That happens often—when the pressure is gone, then people suddenly get pregnant naturally." He means well, I tell myself, I am just oversensitive about it. But what I hear in such encouraging remarks—and I get a number of variations sent my way—is that it is my own fault it is not working. I am trying too hard. I am making things too difficult. I am a neurotic woman with an exaggerated need for a child. If I just stopped trying, it would happen by itself. Just stop! If I knew it would help, there is nothing I would rather do. IVF certainly isn't a hobby of mine.

I also blame myself for things not working. We shouldn't have made love a week after the implant of the embryo. I shouldn't have worked so hard. I shouldn't have drunk any alcohol at all, instead of just the occasional glass.

Paul and I book a week's vacation in the sun on one of the Canary Islands. Holidays are a proven way for us to recover from our disappointments. It is good to be in a different environment and to spoil my tortured body with sun and sea, good food and drink. It is also good for us to consider the future together. We had planned to undertake a maximum of three IVF attempts, and now two of them are behind us. "Three times does the trick," my mother tries to encourage me, but we ourselves see the end drawing nearer with ominous clarity.

During a wine-soaked meal on a terrace overlooking the sea we hold a somber conversation. Paul says that he realizes for the first time that it may all be for nothing. I ask him whether he is thinking of having children with another woman. It had occurred to him that he could do so, he replies. "But the idea of leaving you for that reason is far from my mind," he adds reassuringly.

I don't know what to think of his remark. Generally people do not leave one another for rational reasons. Generally they simply fall in love with someone else if their relationship becomes unsatisfactory, for whatever reason. How long will it be before I hear from him that he is leaving me for another woman, with whom he will then immediately have a child?

No, even worse, I will obviously have to move out, because our house is far too large for me on my own. Paul would continue living there with his new family. I'd go back to the city, into the bars, drink and smoke a lot, become a down-at-heel woman. I find the idea that I could be left for this reason hurtful and humiliating. At the same time I can imagine it happening. In the end, people who want children seek partners who are able to fulfill this wish, whether consciously or unconsciously. But we have more holding us together than this stupid desire for a child! Didn't we promise one another something about "for better or for worse"? Would I leave Paul if he lost his legs, because I so enjoy dancing, riding, and walking with him? Probably not. But I would still be able to do all those things with other people. There the comparison falls apart.

We have many difficult conversations during the vacation. We are aware of the seriousness of the situation. We wonder out loud whether our love will survive this childlessness. We no longer know how we should proceed. But in between our somber conversations and my fits of crying, we play tennis, we swim in the sea, we take nice walks. And we make love and crack jokes. I tell him in a challenging tone that he will never find another woman as nice as me. That by and by he will be saddled with some dumb hag and a dozen screaming brats. Then he'll come and beg me on his bended knees to be his mistress. I will consider your request, I assure him in advance, but I can obviously not make you any promises. Perhaps at the time I will have a new admirer whom I will want to be faithful to, a sensitive romantic with poor little children who embrace me as their new mother.

At the end of the week, we are in a somewhat more optimistic frame of mind. We try to find solutions. Why not a modern variant of the concubine? Perhaps we can find someone mad enough to agree to be a surrogate mother for us. Or why don't we ask Maria, who has in the meantime had a healthy set of twins but has no husband and no money and a house that is far too small, if she would like to come and live with us? Perhaps that would be a tremendous solution all around.

I try to imagine it. I like Maria, and I would probably be able to live together with her well enough. But I imagine it might all go too well between Paul and her and the children; I would surely die of jealousy. Perhaps adoption is an option; then you only have the children coming into your home. All these variations are strange to us, but fantasizing about them gives us a break. It creates the illusion that we can come up with solutions ourselves for what may well be an unsolvable problem.

After this healing week come the repercussions. Paul is rarely around, and when we're out he tries to impress other women. I hardly see him. If he is home, he is self-absorbed and barely touches me. Has he made his decision, now that the options have dawned on him? Is he already moving away from me, and has the hunting season opened?

If it is so easy, if it has happened so quickly, he can damn well get out completely! Let him have the courage to go now, not once he has secured his new lover. Otherwise I will move out! He mustn't think I can't live without him! There are plenty of fish in the sea! I hate him. I miss him. I want him to throw his arms around me and call me his darling, say that he will always stay with me, whatever happens, because he loves me so much that he can't imagine a life without me.

My two former housemates, who were always fairly anti-children, have since also had a baby each, and Nicole is already pregnant with her third. I just sent them each a card. Lois has become pregnant unexpectedly with a third child. It is a minor miracle, after all the trouble they had to go to in order to have the twins. The news does not bring unqualified joy; after all, it is extremely soon after the arrival of the twins. But Simon is proud of his seed, which is apparently not so bad after all. Coquettishly they complain that after the birth they will have to use contraceptives again, when it has been so nice not to have to worry. That they can't drink any alcohol for months again. And that they have to come up with more names.

But the most painful thing is that my contact with Isabel remains so difficult. I miss the familiarity and wonder whether we will ever get it back. We both do our best, but that's as far as it goes. She continues to become more pregnant, I more unstable. I have frequent nightmares in which I am standing alone and am barely able to hold myself upright.

I dream I bump into my housemates and Nicole at a big party at which there is a fireworks display. The first two have flat bellies once more, and Nicole is still pregnant. I walk toward them, but they turn away from me. They are offended because I did not come to visit them after they'd had their babies and had shown no interest in their children.

Suddenly everyone starts to run. I am so deep in thought that I don't realize we are being attacked. I try to join the fleeing mass, but it is already too late. I am trapped. The soldiers want to beat me, but I save myself by saying that I just happened to be walking there, I don't belong with the others, I just came to watch the fireworks. Someone shoves stones and gravel into my vagina as I walk; I only notice when it's already inside and, horrified, clean it out.

A group of soldiers see me with my hand feeling around in my crotch. They are fired up by the sight and hit on the idea of gang-raping me. I run off and hide in a house that is being guarded by police officers. However, the soldiers storm in, kill the policemen, and put on the dead men's uniforms, a sort of purple rain suit with pink plastic shoes.

I also put on a rain suit, so that they'll think I'm one of them, but I forget the plastic shoes and put one of my own moon boots on by mistake. I can't find the other one, and so I limp away with one moon boot and one bare foot. I feel really exposed—they will certainly see that I'm in disguise, and then only half-heartedly. So I go back after all to fetch the plastic shoes.

I get them, but I still feel vulnerable because I don't have a gun. Everyone else is walking around with drawn pistols. People are falling down dead all around me. People are throwing stones. People clamber up, only to be pushed to the ground again. I am terrified but walk on as unconcernedly as possible. I want to survive.

Isabel's child is born. It is a girl. We go at once to see her, in Our Lady Hospital, where I was a few years ago with my ectopic pregnancy. She is lying in exactly the same kind of bed as I did. Suddenly I remember how painful it was after the operation if anyone bumped against my bed. Every little jolt was a real assault. "Don't bump the bed," I warn Paul before we congratulate Isabel and Noam and admire the baby.

It was a difficult delivery; the baby was born by Cesarean. Isabel looks yellow from exhaustion, but has a soft expression in her eyes and laughs in a pleased and incredulous manner at her little girl. Noam is over the moon. Their daughter is doing well.

We stand there awkwardly for a while, moved, confused, and sad. We don't stay long. As we are leaving, we run into Isabel's brother. He was the one who told me after my miscarriage that the loss of an unborn child must also be mourned. I often remember that remark. According to the books there are four phases in the process of mourning. Phase 1: denial. Phase 2: anger. Phase 3: sorrow. Phase 4: acceptance.

I have definitely put Phase 1 behind me. I am alternating between Phases 2 and 3. But at the moment I am deep in Phase 3. Isabel's brother says: "How nice to see you two here! It must be difficult for you to visit the hospital right now." Gratefully I brush his remark aside. Fortunately it is raining outside.

My nerves are shot: We are busy with our third IVF attempt. It is now or never. I am extremely emotional and cannot take much more. Isabel phones to cancel our date for a meal at their place. They would rather spend some time together. Logically. Naturally.

A week later, Paul and I go to drop off our gift, a silver teething ring with the child's name engraved on it. After ten minutes we are sent off, just as we are starting to get ready to leave. It is clear that Isabel is still tired from the delivery, and she is also having problems with anemia. She complains about everything. The Cesarean was a traumatic experience for her. I try unsuccessfully to be understanding. She has a beautiful baby on her lap! Let her moan to another mother rather than to me. She also makes an unsuccessful effort to show some interest in us, by asking if we spend much time riding our bikes in the dunes. Riding? I can hardly move; I have just had my vagina wall punctured.

We are now waiting for the results of the fertilization. For us this is our last chance for a child. But she has something else on her mind. Her mind is not on the world outside but focused entirely inward. In this inner world there is no longer a place for me. Why can't I just get used to it? In the car on the way home, I turn the music up full blast and sit with tears streaming down my cheeks. Paul sits silently next to me and puts his hand on my knee.

As I do every year, I go with my mother to the memorial service for those resisters killed in the Bloemendaal dunes in World War II. We walk there in a silent procession. My brother and his children come, too. Now and then Ruth and Benjamin proudly come and hand their loot over to me—wildflowers they have picked along the side of the road in order to lay on the graves in due course. If I don't have any children of my own, then I'm going to extend my role as an aunt.

A friend of my mother's walks next to me. She's a lovely woman of about fifty, who has not had an easy life. I don't know the details, something to do with the war and serious problems at work. I suddenly notice that she is looking at the children just as tenderly as I. I ask whether she ever wanted children.

"Oh yes, very much," she replies, "but life decided otherwise." After a short pause she summarizes years of sorrow in a few sentences. Pregnant twice, a miscarriage at seven months with the first one, at five months with the second. Then her husband died of cancer. After that, she never met anyone who ignited that spark. I am silenced by all the pain.

At the cemetery I look around. So many people who have lost loved ones. And here I stand with my mother and my brother and my nephew and niece, who are holding my hands tightly. I press kisses on the tops of their heads.

Despite everything, we decide on a fourth and final attempt. I tell myself that we are actually keeping to our original three attempts, because the first try didn't count. The infection meant there was no real chance of success. Since that first time I have been given a preventive antibiotic screen. I also receive a sedative now, because the puncturing is more painful every time. This mild form of sedation does not seem to make much difference. On the contrary, this time the assistants have to be called in to keep me under control. I thrash around, although you're obviously supposed to lie still when they're busy sticking a needle inside you. Afterward I can't sleep or walk for two days. If I go through this again, I will take the advice of the hospital: only under anesthetic. Again? Apparently deep down I'm not convinced that this truly is the last time.

I'm not really sure why I keep at it. Perhaps simply because I am unable to stop myself. We have already put so much energy into this that it becomes more and more difficult to put an end to it. Just as with cars that have problems: The more you have invested in them, the more difficult the decision to get rid of them. Against your better judgment you still take them to the mechanic one last time. Once you are on the medical treadmill, it's not so easy to get off. After every unsuccessful attempt the doctors say that we still belong to the group who have a chance. Fertilization is still occurring, and the embryos are of good quality.

The fact that they are not implanting properly is pure bad luck. It would therefore be a great pity to give up now.

In the meantime I am less and less sure whether I really want a child so much. The desire for a child is controlling my life to an ever greater extent, but at the same time is becoming more and more abstract. To protect myself against disappointment, I try very hard to stop imagining any concrete pictures of a future with children. This creates a slightly unreal atmosphere around my desperate attempts to get pregnant. If I have no idea of what this child will mean to me, why on earth am I trying in the first place?

Joyce gives me the telephone number of a masseur who helps with fertility problems. He restores the disturbed equilibrium in the body, which gives one a greater chance of getting pregnant. I thoroughly enjoy being massaged. As he works, he talks about opening up the blockages in my body. As far as I'm aware, I have only one blockage, the one in my Fallopian tubes. I am far too levelheaded for this type of thing, but I willingly allow myself to be kneaded by him.

The embryos are once again of excellent quality. "You haven't had them this good before," the doctors on the IVF team say enthusiastically. There are four embryos. Usually they put a maximum of two back, to reduce the number of multiple births. But the more embryos that are put back, the greater the chances that one or two will make it. I am quite happy with the idea of twins or triplets; then I will get it all over with at once. Four at once does seem a bit much, but it is better than nothing.

"Put all four back, please," I ask, almost pleading. "This is my last attempt. I want to go for broke."

They give in. All the embryos are put into my womb. Once again two long weeks of waiting and hoping start. My father comes by to lay hands on the embryos. By placing his hands on my belly, he tries to encourage the implanting. I feel a little uncomfortable about it, but I also find it very sweet of him. Even if it doesn't help, it can't do any harm.

The fourth attempt fails as well. I feel old and tired of life. We are on a dead-end road. For far too long I have been living from one cycle to the next, from one attempt to the next, from one pregnancy test to the next, from one disappointment to the next. I try as best I can to keep going with everything, but I'm just about at the end of my tether. I almost always plan the numerous hospital visits for before work. This means getting up at the crack of dawn, always feeling rushed and concerned that things may go wrong and I'll be late. And at the same time, I'm trying my best not to get stressed, because stress doesn't seem to be good for a solid implantation.

I put everything on hold, because all future plans are influenced by a possible pregnancy. Making serious work of a new job? I can't. After another unsuccessful attempt, I have too little motivation to make a good impression in a job interview; I am too sad and too tired, I am not focused enough. When I have gathered together enough energy for a further IVF effort, the chance of success holds me back from undertaking anything new. What if I get pregnant? Being pregnant when you are starting a new job doesn't seem right to me. As it is, I am not going to have a nice, relaxed pregnancy. If I have to immerse myself in a new job at the same time, I will probably have a miscarriage from the stress. Go away on a long trip? What if I get pregnant and have complications while I'm away in Africa?

I must stop this. I can't keep it up. I want to leave, the sooner the better. I want to have adventures that will put new life into me. I want my future back.

We decide to extend a planned business trip to Mexico and take a long vacation together. Our desire for a child was born seven years ago in America. America is the land of dreams. Mexico is the land of the dead. It is a good place to bury desire.

CHAPTER SEVEN

THE END,

or

The Laying of the Last Egg

I am late. I had my last period six weeks ago. I blame it on my hormones, which are probably confused after all the IVF attempts. Because we're leaving for Mexico in a week, I want to know what's going on. So I decide to do a pregnancy test. Positive. Pregnant. I think of my brother's words. Could it be true that you get pregnant as soon as you stop trying? I phone the hospital immediately and am able to go the same day for an ultrasound. The screen shows an empty uterus. Stay calm. It needn't mean anything. Perhaps it's still too early in the pregnancy to see anything. The blood test will decide.

The intern is a nicely made-up young lady, with the high-spirited haughtiness of someone on whom life has not yet left its mark. She is practicing to be a doctor; I am a practiced patient. I tell her that I may have an ectopic pregnancy and that I have been referred to this hospital near where I live in case an emergency admission becomes necessary. In the tone of a nursery school teacher, she starts going through her list of questions. She keeps recording my answers incorrectly. I watch her and correct her. I know my file by heart. The medical encyclopedia has become my favorite book. I am the type of person who likes to know and understand everything. It gives me the feeling of having some control over the situation, and I need this now more than ever. So I fire my questions at her: "If the embryo is in the left Fallopian tube, will they remove the whole thing?" And: "If they remove my left Fallopian tube, could they do something about the blockage in the right one during the operation?"

She has just one clincher available to her: "We'll look at all that when we plan to operate." I give up and leave to have some blood taken. According to the intern the results will be available on Monday. It is now Friday. It will be a difficult weekend, waiting in suspense.

At the counter I happen to hear that the blood test results will, in fact, be available in a few hours' time. I am annoyed that the Barbie doll wanted to make me wait unnecessarily until Monday. The result is reassuring. We don't need to worry about having to be admitted over the weekend.

On Monday morning I have to have more blood taken and make another appointment. On the advice of my general practitioner, I insist on being able to speak to the treating doctor myself. After I have waited a good hour, the doctor finally appears, a man who gives the impression of being rather absentminded.

Once again I explain the situation. I tell him about my previous history, the last operation, my attempts at IVF. Because he looks impatient, I cut my explanations short and ask my questions again, as concisely as possible.

His answers are short and sharp. "Yes" to the question of whether the whole left Fallopian tube will be removed if the embryo is developing in it. "It then becomes a 'tomy.'"

"A what?"

"An abdominal operation."

To the question of whether something can be done to the right Fallopian tube at the same time the answer is: "No." In the meantime the results of the blood test come in. There is such an incredibly high level of pregnancy hormones in my blood that the gynecologist suspects it may not be an ectopic pregnancy after all, but a normal one. A new ultrasound must be done. Hope flickers. It's all been a bad joke, to test me. My patience will soon be rewarded. I will turn out to have an ordinary pregnancy, and in the end everything will be okay.

Waiting in the waiting room again. The waiting is always the worst. Finally it is my turn. Tense, I watch the screen during the ultrasound. I am looking for movement, a beating heart. The screen only shows a grey amorphous mass. Not a single sign of life.

Another ectopic pregnancy. Another emergency admission. We have to cancel the trip to Mexico. Life is playing a game with me. Let's see how far I can go with you. You still think that you have everything in control. That you can plan and determine your own future. I have not yet managed to beat the pride out of you. I will still teach you a lesson in humility.

I am only allowed to go home quickly to fetch my things. Nervously I call a few friends and members of the family. I hear myself reproaching Isabel and my sister-in-law, who hadn't phoned to find out how things were going. The same old song. I expect too much sympathy, I must stop this. When will I grow up?

We hurry. We needn't have bothered. When we get back, I have to wait hours before I am given a bed. Hours after that an intern arrives and has to set up a drip. He makes an absolute hash of it, as if it is his first time. He first tries on the left, but just can't get it right. When my arm is so full of holes that it is starting to become inflamed, he moves to the right.

"If it doesn't work this time, they'll have to fire me," he laughs. It doesn't work again, and he disappears from sight, probably to get his letter of dismissal.

Another hour later—it's now eleven at night—a doctor is finally available. They've moved me, bed and all, to an examination room so that the other five women in the ward can go to sleep without being disturbed. What a relief. When the drip is finally set up, I ask the doctor whether I may stay there for the night. I may. I have a thick book with me about life in the ghetto in Warsaw, which I read all night long. It is so gripping and moving that I forget where I am and why.

But in the morning my book is finished and I am taken back to the ward. I want to be alone; I don't want to hear what the others are going to be operated on for, or why they have already been operated on. One of the nurses notices my state and asks whether she should phone someone for me. Her tone is so kind that I can no longer keep my tears back. She closes the curtain around my bed, so I have at least a degree of privacy, and phones Paul, who appears to be on his way already.

He comes and sits on the edge of my bed and doesn't leave until my mother arrives. She is even more nervous about the operation than I am but tries not to show it and talks incredibly fast. Her torrent of words has a calming effect on me.

Then she is sent away, too. My pubic hair has to be shaved. I am as bald as a newly plucked chicken. Over time I have become familiar with these preparatory rituals. Take all clothes off, hand in watch and rings, put on a sterile hospital gown and a little cap. In a few minutes the metamorphosis of individual to patient is complete once again.

When I come to in the recovery room, the first thing I ask is: "Was it a laparoscopy or a tomy?"—as if I am the doctor rather than the patient. An abdominal operation, is the answer. That means: My only good Fallopian tube is gone. That means: I will never be able to get pregnant naturally again. That means: an ugly scar right across my abdomen, just as with a

Cesarean, but without the reward of a child. That means they had to cut right through my abdominal muscles and that it will take far longer to recover than last time. I start crying softly, but soon stop, because any movement is painful.

God bless the inventor of painkillers. They mute everything. I am allowed to go back to my own examining room, where Paul is already waiting for me. He holds my hand tightly and is very loving toward me. He also has become practiced. Later my mother and Isabel and Noam arrive. I am very glad to see them. It is as if I have been resurrected from the dead and returned to the land of the living.

My mother suddenly notices that the drip is empty. We call someone in, who figures out that it has been empty for some time. A new one will have to be attached. Once again a lot of clumsy and painful fiddling with my arm. It annoys me enormously, all this poking and prodding with my body. Because I so want to be alone, I am allowed to stay and sleep in the examining room again.

I come to regret this during the night. At my request they put me near the intercom so that I can call someone if I need to. I keep waking up with a fright to check my drip. And just in time, too. I feel for the intercom, which requires a code to start working. It is so dark in the room that I can't find the code. There is no way I can get the thing talking.

In the meantime the all-powerful drip changes roles: I am no longer being given any liquid; instead my blood is slowly being sucked into the little tube. How long will it take for the plastic bag to be filled with my blood? How much blood can a person do without? I start to call, but my voice is still hoarse from the anesthetic. No one hears me.

I think of the story of my Aunt Ingrid, who was put in an empty room "just for a while" after an operation. She was remembered only a day and a half later, when some visitors arrived for her.

In a panic I start to cry and scream, but then I tell myself to be calm. I must save my voice for when I hear someone walking past.

Eventually someone hears me. I get a new drip, and a flashlight. After that I don't sleep a wink. I am fixated on my drip. It fills my mind completely. And it is as if the Devil is in it: The next one also runs dry without anyone coming to check. This time I am able to call a nurse on the intercom. I tell her angrily that this is the third drip that they have forgotten to come and replace. They don't have to do anything else with me, except make sure that the damn thing is replaced in time so that I don't have to worry about it. As it is, I have a sleep-less night and an operation behind me. I would like to be able to sleep peacefully. I expect an excuse, but the nurse looks sullen and doesn't say a word. Another hysterical patient tak-ing her frustrations out on me, I can see her thinking.

The next day Dr. De Koning comes to my bedside for the postoperative discussion. "I left your right Fallopian tube in, although it would have been better to remove it, because if both Fallopian tubes have been removed the chances of success with IVF are greater," he says. From my horrified reaction I realize that I haven't yet given up completely on IVF. More than ever, it is my last chance now.

I ask the doctor why he didn't remove the right Fallopian tube as well.

"I can't do that without permission. We didn't discuss it beforehand," he replies.

I can't believe my ears. He is using his own lack of interest as an excuse! "So why didn't you ask whether I would agree?" I say as he once again starts getting ready to move on to the next bed.

"Oh, it is always so emotional," he mumbles before taking off. Psychiatrists have to undergo counseling as part of their training. They should make other doctors undergo surgery as part of theirs.

I give myself up to the slow rhythm of recovery. A drip brings fluid into my body, a catheter carries it away. Gradually I reclaim my body from the apparatus. Paul lovingly massages my head, which seems about to burst from pain, probably as a result of the anesthetic. When the worst of the pain has passed, I start to look forward longingly to visiting hours. What

I would really like is to have people around me for every minute of that time. But talking and listening are tiring. If there are several people there, they sometimes also talk to one another, or over one another. And they all move so much. From one minute to the next, my joy at their presence turns into irritation and an exhausted desire for rest.

My senses are not yet able to take in all the stimuli. When, after a week in the hospital, Paul takes me in the car, I look around foolishly. How fast the cars are driving! Everyone is in such a hurry. I feel assaulted by the noisiness and all the movement in the outside world. Even in my own house I am not safe: The neighbors are busy hammering. I long for the quiet, white world of the hospital. When I start crying, I can't stop. Paul phones my mother. She comes at once and with unusual tenderness wipes the wet streaks from my face. Her comforting gesture has a restful effect. "Hello, my dear daughter," she says. "Cry if you want to; it hasn't been easy for you." She stays sitting next to me until I drift into sleep.

I lie in the bath and immerse myself in the water to the sound of Yiddish songs, which I haven't listened to for a long time because Paul finds it so sentimental. The hot water opens my pores, through which the melancholy sounds penetrate right into me. When I am not lying in the bath, I lie in bed and read a book about the soul, which my father gave me as a present. Normally I would have put it on the shelf, untouched. I am always too busy with things of this world. Not now, though; now I have all the time in the world. I don't have to do anything. I don't have to make any decisions. I exist and endure.

After a few days I take my first shaky walk around the block on my friend Anna's arm, scared that someone might knock me over or bump my stomach. It is a foretaste of the brittleness of old age. But I get stronger every day. Every day I walk a little farther.

A week later I make it to the pharmacy on my own, where I buy not only cream for my scar but also makeup, bath oil, and body lotion. Comfort for my body. The last time, my abdomen was sore for a good six months after the operation because I did not take care of myself. Now I am wiser. My body and I have to travel on together; we need to be good to one another.

My mother and I trade places. I have only just left the hospital when she has to go in. She has a tumor in the head. The swelling is the size of an egg. What is it with eggs that they settle themselves in places in our bodies where they do not belong? My mother has always had a lot of trouble with headaches. "My tumor is playing up again," she would sigh. In retrospect an apt joke. The doctors say that it is probably benign, can be operated on, and, if everything goes well, will heal well.

It's one thing for them to be so positive. She is in a panic. She has never had an operation, and now the first time she does, they want to open up her skull and cut inside! What she finds the worst is that they are going to shave her head before the operation. A shaved head precedes death. Her mother, her aunts, her nieces and nephews were all shaved in the war.

I take her to a smart shop to buy her a nice hat before the operation. The outing is a nerve-racking mission to exorcise the fear. Neither of us has ever bought a hat before. We behave like rowdy teenagers having a joke at the expense of the shop assistant.

"Do you have something that will sit nicely on a bare white head?" asks my mother with a straight face when it is our turn. "It's not a present, it's for myself." Screaming with laughter we try on almost every hat in the shop.

"We're actually looking for a magician's hat," I explain when the assistant tries to find out just what it is we want. "It doesn't need to have doves coming out of it. One egg will be enough for us." We double up again, while the shop assistant puckers her eyebrows helplessly. We choose an expensive hat, which helps to put things right.

Dying is bad, but still preferable to serious brain damage. We talk about degrees: what is acceptable, what not. It feels absurd to talk about acceptance when none of us knows the extent of this unpleasant adventure. Still these conversations have to be held now. Shortly before the operation she asks me if I will sign a euthanasia statement to be used in the event that she is no longer in control of her faculties. My hand shakes as I sign. It is as if I am signing her death warrant in advance. She has made a will. She gives me her bank number so that in an emergency I have access to her account. She tells me where her valuables are kept. She shows me an album that she has kept up-to-date for her eldest granddaughter, with photos and information about our family history. Her neat, regular writing moves me. She seldom talks about the past, but on these pages she has laid it out in detail for future generations.

I wish that I could also have given her a grandchild. I want to say something to her, something I still have the chance to do, before it perhaps becomes too late. I want to thank her for everything she has done for me. I want to tell her how much I love her. But by doing that I would be underlining my signature on her death warrant. So I give her a kiss and say: "There is no way you can die. You are far too lively for that." She nods obediently, like a trusting child.

She is completely bald and lies hooked up to all sorts of alarming machines. But she is alive. Anxiously she asks: "How bald am I?"

THE END

| 127 |

"Completely bald, but the work has been done, the egg has been laid."

She lets out a breath and says triumphantly: "Then I am the first in our family to have survived a bald head."

After one visit I stand in the parking lot talking to my eldest brother's wife. The family ties have been drawn tighter through concern about my mother. Suddenly my sister-in-law says: "I am so sorry that you are not having any luck with having children. I would so like you to be able to, you would be such great parents. Our family is now complete. If it would help you, I am willing to carry a child for you."

I see that she means it and am silent in the face of such a generous offer. I cannot accept it. She is no longer all that young, and I know how difficult her last delivery was. But I am eternally grateful to her for this huge gesture.

After the first sense of relief follows a week of waiting for the results: Did they remove the tumor completely or not, is it benign or malignant? Even my father sits shaking with nervousness in the waiting room. At the appointed time no result is available; the next day still nothing is known. My mother is suffering like the bridge of a violin under strings that are stretched too tightly. She stays lying in bed, doesn't want to talk anymore, to eat anything, to wash herself. All she can do is cry. If you are waiting for what might well be your death sentence, you cling to the only certainty you have: the moment at which you will receive the decision. It is extremely cruel to take that certainty away from someone as well. I am furious with the nonchalant doctor, who doesn't even take the trouble to explain the reason for the delay.

Days later, when we have virtually given up hope, he finally comes in with a serious look on his face. "The scar is looking healthy," he says as he peers with an indiscreet gesture under the bandage that covers my mother's bald head. I look at the unfamiliar landscape of bumps and dents, which looks as if an inexperienced potter has been working with a lump of clay. "Once the hair has grown out a bit, you won't even see it," he says reassuringly, as if that is our greatest concern at the moment. Get a move on, man. If it is malignant, damn well tell us and don't keep us in suspense any longer. At last it comes out: "It was a benign tumor. We were able to remove the whole thing."

The operation was completely successful. My mother will recover! Crying, we embrace one another. I have been walking around with a bottle of champagne in my bag for days, in anticipation of this moment. Now we can pop the cork. Lechaim! To life!

They say that you learn from difficult experiences. I always wonder what you gain from these lessons. It is a lot more pleasant to be saved from them. They simply turn you gray before your time. Wise, they call it. But disaster is disaster. Loss is loss. You have to deal with it; there's no other choice. Anyone who says that loss is actually gain, that it enriches you, is turning things around. But I have to concede that my mother's life is pure gain. Also for me. Not only because I did not lose her, when it was a near thing, but also because I was able to forget my own troubles. And now it has all worked out okay. It has been a long time since I have been able to be really glad for someone else. It is as if I am at last allowed outside, after a long period of being shut up alone.

Now I become aware of what I have always known at the back of my mind: that my situation isn't all that bad. I will soon be my old self; I am getting better by the day. My setbacks have not had a fundamental effect on my health, as a malignant tumor would. A tumor can poison your life from one day to the next. With a little bad luck it simply stops and you die. Perhaps I won't have any children, but I am healthy and I am alive.

I no longer have to keep track of when I am fertile and when I should be starting a period. No more pregnancy tests for me if I am a few days late. No more folic acid tablets, which I have been taking every day for years to prevent a miscarriage. I have been released from the hope of a spontaneous pregnancy.

Only IVF remains a possibility. But I can determine its timing myself, and I can also decide against it. Someone who has been missing for years and does not return is declared dead at a certain point, so that those remaining behind, who cannot keep on hoping forever, can move on. Because I was exhausted by the IVF attempts, I have decided to bury my desire for a child. We did not need to travel to the land of the dead to do it. Death thrust itself upon us via my mother's tumor, in the form of an egg. But we have escaped the dance.

The scar on my abdomen fades slowly, and the scar on my mother's head disappears under her new hair. She no longer has to wear the magician's hat. Later she tells me that my younger sister is expecting her third child. My sister was afraid to tell me herself. I phone to congratulate her. The fit of crying that generally follows this type of call does not come.

Delighted with this new milestone, I phone Isabel. "I'd like to see you. Shall we go out somewhere?" There is silence on the other end of the line. "I'll treat you to a nice meal, and we'll drink like we used to do," I add.

"Yes, that's a very good idea," she says softly. "Let's do that. Then we can finally catch up with one another."

Paul and I ask my eleven-year-old niece Ruth to come and stay. The three of us ride our bikes down to the beach and roll from the top of a sand dune down to the bottom. Elated, we run down to the sea. After our walk on the beach, we go and have lunch in a cafe. We eat toasted sandwiches and drink hot chocolate with whipped cream. Like a woman of the world, Ruth looks around her. She seldom goes into a restaurant. "Do you know what I like so much about you two?" she asks in a charming conspiratorial tone. She looks penetratingly at Paul and me in turn; she is about to entrust us with something important.

"What?" I ask curiously.

"You are such fun. My parents are much stricter."

"If we were your parents, we would also be much stricter," says Paul, as strictly as he can.

My niece doesn't believe him.

I have plucked up my courage. I am just not certain what type of courage: the courage to do something or the courage to turn away. I feel I have the strength of someone who has survived a natural disaster. They will not get me down again. I could have a repair operation to clear the blockage in my remaining Fallopian tube, even though the chances of success are relatively small. I could undergo one last IVF treatment. But I could also leave it. If I have to give up, then this is the right time. I believe that I am strong enough to deal with my loss. We have done our best. It has been good. It is now time for the fat years to begin.

Paul does not want to see me lying in a hospital bed with a white face and a battered belly again. He says that he can now accept that we will not be having any children, but first he would like to investigate seriously the possibility of adopting. He is getting near the legal age limit for adopting a baby. No one in our circle of friends has adopted a child. I associate adoption with problem cases. I don't want to be a do-gooder; I simply want a child or, if necessary, no child. I loathe the idea of being obliged to do a course, to go onto a waiting list, to be screened for my suitability as a parent, even though it appears to be a mere formality. I tell myself that people who adopt are generally really motivated parents, with a far deeper-seated desire for a child than ours.

On the other hand, why shouldn't we actually do it? Why is it so necessary for us to have a child of our own flesh? That is no guarantee against problems. Adoption also has something adventurous about it. I like adventures. Such a procedure involves shuffling papers, not manipulating your body. It requires time and patience, but in between you can do what you like. At the end of the whole procedure, there is a 100 percent chance of having a child. This is a far higher success rate than with IVF.

At a party I get into a conversation with a woman who has adopted two children. She says it was the best decision she ever made. "How did you make it?" I ask curiously.

"I wanted to have a child in my arms very much," she says. The simplicity of her argument strikes me. That's also how it was for me when I asked Paul for the first time whether we should make a baby. What has remained of that simple wish for a child?

We give ourselves a trip to South Africa to sort out our thoughts. It has been a number of years since we last took a trip to a far-off destination together. The last one was to Guatemala and Honduras. I came back from that trip with my plan to have a tattoo, in an effort to gain control over the desire for a child. Now I am hoping we will come back with a decision about letting it go.

We meet an elderly backpacking couple. They have no children but take the most wonderful trips around the world. We see ourselves in twenty years' time. It is not an unattractive picture. From our comfortable lodgings with a sea view, we go through all the destinations on our wish list.

The guesthouse is run by a balding man with a cap and an inextinguishable entrepreneurial spirit. His first business had been a "Rent a Husband" service. He had meant it in all innocence as a handyman business, but the name created other expectations, and it expanded to become an escort service for women. But he found success boring. Whenever anything was running well, he started something else. We spend the night with him, drinking and listening to his endless stories. His work is his food and drink. Fired up by his enthusiasm, we start dreaming about the types of businesses we could start. One plan bubbles up after the next. Anything is possible.

Next to where we are staying lives a small black boy, about four years old, with big shiny mischievous eyes. He is always playing in the street, where we see him at least twice a day—in the morning, when we set out hand in hand down the road to go for a walk or to take a dip in the sea, and in the evening when we come back, tired and content. We always play the same little game with him. "Hello, mister!" Paul calls out to him and puts out his hand politely as if he is greeting a very important person.

"Hello, mister!" the boy replies gleefully as he takes Paul's hand and starts to shake it so hard that his arm almost comes out of its socket. Paul brings his left arm up to his right shoulder and with a grimace of pain falls moaning to the ground. Together we try to get him on his feet again, each on one arm, which is not at all easy, since we are laughing ourselves sick. The little boy has an infectious laugh. I imagine what it would be like if he was our child. The idea becomes less and less strange.

Nature here is enormously spread out. There is no one to be seen all around us. We take off all our clothes and run into the sea. The waves are exactly how I like them best: high but regular. They don't break just before the shore, but quite a way back in the sea, and then roll onto the beach. The trick is to be just in front at the moment that the wave breaks. Then the upper current takes you with it, and you become one with the white ridges, which carry you along on their powerful backs. You just have to surrender yourself and enjoy it.

"Now!" I shout to Paul as the moment to dive comes around again. Sometimes he stays behind, sometimes he's in front of me, but just once we come out together at the same place. Paul's eyes are glittering with enjoyment. I still find him extremely attractive. He has a slim but athletic body that shines brown and wet in the sun. We wallow in the warm sand and peer at the blue water.

Suddenly we see something moving out there. It is some dolphins, which jump up out of the waves and then dive back in. Neither of us has ever seen real dolphins before. Rhythmically they move up and down, with a wonderful elasticity and suppleness. We jump up in order to see them better. There are a whole lot of them. Every time we think the last one has disappeared from sight, new elegant curves appear on the horizon.

"May I make an indecent proposal?" I ask Paul ecstatically. "Shall we take another plunge?"

EPILOGUE

A lot has happened since this book first came out in the original Dutch edition. Of course I had hoped the book would find its way to the readers, but I could never have dreamed that it would reach so many. It became a best seller in the Netherlands and was sold in eighteen countries in and outside of Europe. I was invited to countries such as Spain, Finland, and South Africa to do interviews about the book. I received emotional and heartwarming reactions from readers all over the world, mostly women, sometimes men, telling me their own life stories and thanking me for the support the book had given them. For me, it proves the power of words and the possibility to share experiences and find comfort in them. I find this incredibly rewarding.

Many readers have asked me how the story of my life continued. Quite happily I can say that our two daughters, whom we adopted as babies, are seven and nine years old now, and they are doing very well. They are very conscious of their background and ask a lot of questions about their birth country. At the end of this year, we will visit Guatemala for the first time as a family. My mother is healthy, alive, and kicking and

138

plays an important role in the lives of my daughters. Paul is still the love of my life and a wonderful father to our daughters. Sadly his father and brother have died in the meantime, but we are still close to Gwen, who is a wonderful grandmother to both our children and her daughter's three wild boys. Isabel is still my best friend, and my children love to play with hers. Every year we spend our holidays all together. My professional life has also further developed, and I became a publisher of a prestigious literary house in Amsterdam. The only thing lacking in my life now is the time to write more books. But I promise you, one day I will!

Judith Uyterlinde

REACTIONS FROM READERS

The life of this book is a story in itself. In the space of a few years, it has been published in eighteen countries and found more than three hundred thousand readers around the world. Since then Judith has received thousands of letters from readers, extracts of which are below. If you would also like to write to the author, send an email to editorial@GlobePequot.com, and we will forward it to her.

Certain books grab you from the very first line. That is the case with this one. I read it in one go and when I put it down, I was stunned. I immediately bought three copies: two for friends and one for my sister. Not to reproach them: "See what I have been through and how badly you reacted!" It was to give them the gift of a moving book, full of humor, that tells of the ordeal that so many women have lived through.

Michaela

I congratulate you on the way you describe your emotions. It truly took my breath away, something I have never experienced with any other book. Never before have I read passages that seem to come straight from my own heart. Your book helps us to live with the suffering that haunts us, and shows us the way to happiness.

Annette

As a gynecologist, I recommend your book ten times a week to numerous couples who are following the same path that you have taken. I am sorry for the insensitive reactions of the doctors that you met, who were not aware of the impact of their words. My colleagues should all read your book so that they can understand their patients.

Helen

My wife and I tried for years to have a child and finally resorted to IVF treatment. We failed. Finally, in 2002, we adopted our little Korean boy, even though we had never previously considered adoption. I am not much of a reader, but I came upon your book by chance and I read it in one go because it told our story: the lack of understanding of family and friends— I recognized everything that had happened to us.

Peter

You have done what should have been done a long time ago: write a book about the deep pain caused by infertility, which unfortunately affects more and more couples. You have given those going through this ordeal the ability to talk more easily with their family and friends about what is happening to them. Because it is of utmost importance that those around us understand what we feel when the child that we want so much doesn't come.

Herma

It is an incredible book. My sister-in-law tried in vain to have a child and this book has helped me to understand what she was experiencing. Now it is easier to talk about it. Thank you for this personal account.

Jacqueline

From now on, when it comes to birthdays, I will no longer have to rack my brains to think of what to give my friends— the ones who give you advice with the best intentions in the world but do nothing more than drive the knife into the wound. Thank you for this sincere personal account which is full of humor.

Petra

Thank you for writing such a sincere book. I myself am the father of two children. But amongst our friends, several couples are facing the problem that you describe. Your book has helped me and my wife to understand better the ordeal that they are going through, to understand better what they are feeling, and to react better, which isn't always easy when you don't know much about this problem. I will certainly recommend this book to those around me. Few men are open to this sort of personal account. For my own part, I am very grateful to you for allowing me to understand what a woman feels in such a situation.

Jim

I loved your book. My husband and I have a seven-year-old daughter. But we would like a second child and after three miscarriages, five attempts at intrauterine insemination and two IVF treatments, I still have not conceived. I completely recognized myself in your story. The emotions that you describe are so real. I admire you for finally coming to terms with this ordeal and choosing adoption.

Maria

It was very moving, familiar, and funny at times too—a fantastic book, and brilliantly written.

Jet

For me, your book brought lots of buried emotions to the surface. I bought it on the recommendation of a friend—who has been through the same ordeal—and I read it in a few hours. I really appreciate the frankness with which you describe your emotions. Your book is captivating and remarkably sincere. It's a real delight to read, even if the emotions which it provokes are extremely painful. I spent an hour crying in the shower and then I picked up a pen myself and started to write about my unfulfilled desire for a child, which ended up destroying my relationship. The ordeal of medical treatments was, however, successful for us. I gave birth to twins, who are now three years old. The father of my children left me after the fourth failure to have a third child. I am now alone with my twins. They fill me with happiness, but it's not quite the life that I dreamed of. I have ended up accepting, little by little, everything that has happened to me and your book is a great support to me. Thank you.

Mary

Thank you for your book. Few books have touched me so deeply. I recognized my own story in it, my own emotions. It could have been my book. Thank you infinitely.

Rosanna

I bought your book on Thursday afternoon and by the same evening I had finished it. I couldn't put it down. It's a wonderful book! I had already read quite a bit about infertility, but what you wrote really came from the heart. You have described so well what you feel when you are denied the one thing you desire most in the world. I am thirty-three. For three years my husband and I have been trying for a child. We are soon to undergo IVF treatment. I wish you much happiness and thank you for this personal account.

Jolanda

I have just read your book and it confronted me once again with all the emotions that I felt when I was in the same situation: the despair, the doubt, the anger. It all resurfaced.

Monique

Thank you for writing this book. I saw myself in it straight away. I knew well enough that I wasn't the only one going through this, but I was unaware that we all have the same thoughts, the same emotions: the sense of loneliness during a meal with friends, the ambivalence that you feel when your friends get pregnant, of which you feel a little ashamed. I completely recognized myself in what you wrote. I am going to give your book to all of my friends.

Herma

Deeply moving, the way in which you have written my story!

Eva

I want you to know that I read your book in one go. It cost me a whole box of tissues, which doesn't detract from the fact that I thought it was wonderful, and all too familiar.

Tina

In 1986 I attempted my first IVF treatment, without success. My husband and I finally decided to adopt a child, as you have done. Reading this book made all the sadness I felt at that time resurface. This book is a tremendous support for all the couples who don't succeed in having children, but above all for those close to them. I wanted to show you my gratitude for having put down on paper everything that I felt, but was incapable of expressing.

Ria

I really saw myself in this book. It was my story. I will explain to you briefly: two miscarriages, two ectopic pregnancies, five IVF treatments, a hemorrhage and, like you, drips that hospital staff forgot to refill (incredible, no?), the anxiety, and loneliness of nights spent in hospital. I want to know how you feel now. . . . What happens when you finally give up. . . . I love the way the book ends.

Dorine

READING GROUP GUIDE

1. At the very beginning of her narrative, Judith Uyterlinde makes the comment "I figure that having children is part of living." What do you think of this statement? Do you agree or disagree? Do you believe that you can have a complete, fulfilling life without children?

2. On page 4, Judith remarks that she "no longer saw living with a man as robbing me of my freedom" in reference to her relationship to Paul. Do you believe that the *right* relationship never limits our independence—or, do you think that any long-term relationship ultimately includes some form of compromise?

3. What do you think of the idea of making love to "banish the specter of death"? Do you think that in moments of crisis we are drawn to physical intimacy?

4. Why do you think Judith includes the section about Dick's stroke and his hospital stay? Do you think this foreshadows Judith's own future disappointment?

5. On page 7, Judith notes that she mentions her pregnancy to everyone because it makes it more *real* to her. Do you find that sharing personal milestones with others does the same for you? Do you think this is also true of sharing bad news? Do you ever avoid sharing bad news keep it from becoming fully real, or do you find that it helps you to talk about it?

6. The one place Judith fails to discuss her initial pregnancy is at work. How do women have to navigate issues of pregnancy in the workplace? Have you ever been fearful of telling a boss that you were pregnant, or worried that your company might be displeased if you became pregnant? Do you see a divide between "pregnant women" and "career women"?

7. What did you think about the scene (starting on page 12) where Judith has a miscarriage? Given that she didn't feel well, do you think that Paul should have remained home with her? Were you annoyed that he didn't?

8. Were you struck by the juxtaposition of the cold, clinical language of the doctors (using words such as "fetal matter" and "material") with Judith's raw, emotional heartache?

9. On page 65, Judith remarks, "I cannot free myself of my shackles, because it is my own body that has for the second time given me such a raw deal." What can you do when the

popular methods of escape no longer work, when you cannot free yourself from the limits of your own body? Have you ever felt hindered by your body in any way?

10. After Judith suffers an ectopic pregnancy, she immerses herself in renovating their new house, finding a measure of relief in this sort of intense, physical activity. How do you cope with emotional disappointment? What sorts of activities or distractions help you to alleviate feelings of frustration and depression?

11. Isabel's pregnancy clearly puts a strain on her friendship with Judith. Do you think she had a right to be irritated with Judith for being so self-absorbed, or do you think that she failed to acknowledge the depth of Judith's grief? Who did you sympathize with? What are some other large issues that can test a friendship?

12. When Judith travels to the Frankfurt book fair, she encounters a literary agent who believes that women have been "programmed" by men to want children. What did you think of this provocative statement? Do you think this is possible, or do you believe that it is a natural desire? How much influence does nature have versus culture?

13. What are your thoughts on In Vitro Fertilization (IVF)? Do you think that it's a valuable option for women who have

difficulty conceiving? Can it become dangerous—both physi-
cally and emotionally—when a woman repeatedly turns to IVF,
even when it fails to work? Does it make it hard to set limits
and stick to them because of the temptation to simply try *one
more time*?

14. Judith talks about how people often become compet-
itive about the extent of their suffering. Do you have friends,
family, or coworkers who are like this? How does it make you
feel? Do you ever find yourself falling into this behavior? Do
you ever find it difficult to align your "heart" with your "mind"?
How can you respond more appropriately and compassion-
ately to someone else's suffering?

15. Why do you think it took her mother's tumor and brain
surgery to snap Judith out of her own misery?

16. What did you think of the book's ending? Did you find it
hopeful? Do you think that traveling to new places can help you
to leave the past behind and find peace? Do you think that her
interaction with the four-year-old boy in South Africa enabled
Judith to more fully explore the possibility of adoption?

17. Is adoption a solution to infertility? Can it heal the
wounds of being infertile? Can it be as satisfying as biological
motherhood?

ACKNOWLEDGMENTS

Thanks to my two daughters from Guatemala, and to the love of my life, without whom I wouldn't have been able to write this book. To my mother, who is there when I need her. My father, who always supports me. My best friend, with whom I can now survive all storms. My other beloved family members and friends, especially Erika Heppner who can now read my book in English. My sweet Dutch publishers Jan, Maarten, and Pleun. My dear friend and agent Anna Soler-Pont, who, with the help of Marina Penalva-Halpin, sold this book in so many countries. All of my foreign publishers who took the trouble to work on the translations of my book and made it have so many new lives. A special thanks to Mary Norris, Lara Asher, and their other colleagues at skirt!, who have worked with so much devotion on the U.S. edition you now have in your hands. I am really happy and proud that the book has traveled this far and has now reached you.

ABOUT THE AUTHOR

Judith Uyterlinde studied Spanish literature and translation science. She worked as a translator at the European Union in Brussels and as a literary critic for *NRC*, a Dutch daily newspaper and for *Onzewereld*, a monthly magazine. From 1990 onwards she worked as an acquiring editor of foreign literature for various Dutch publishing houses and was publisher of Meulenhoff, a literary house in Amsterdam. She now devotes her time to writing books and articles. Judith was born in Bennebroek, a small village in the Dutch flower region, and lives with her husband and two adopted daughters in Overveen, not far from Amsterdam and close to the sea.

FINALLY!

A skirt that fits!

SKIRT MAGAZINE.